SUPERFOODS
FOR SPORT PERFORMANCE

BUILD YOUR DIETARY ROUTINE

ANDY GRIMM

Summary

1.

NUTRITION, HEALTH AND SPORTS PERFORMANCE

....

"Diet is like a game strategy. You have to plan it carefully to get the most out of yourself."

Novak Djokovic

This book was born from a simple idea: to have a game plan... at the table, focusing your attention on certain pieces in particular, some foods that - as we will see - have been defined as super, certainly sparking interest for those who love to perform and approach life as a constant challenge.

The greatest champions in sports learn this among the first rudiments of their careers: choosing the right foods is a key factor in achieving and maintaining success. Just like the effort during training, but with the advantage that eating correctly is also rewarding (and often less demanding than a five-hour workout in the sun). Whether you're a professional athlete or a fitness and sports enthusiast in general, like myself, with this small volume, you will learn to consider some foods as an integral part of your daily preparation, your strategy.

Proper nutrition will not only allow you to perform better, endure, and recover more effectively after each workout, but also to feel better in your body, day by day, achieving and, above all, maintaining your best physical shape without extreme choices.

Think of it this way: your training routine doesn't just involve exercises and breaks, sets and recoveries, distances and repetitions. Your training routine also includes the proper selection of foods. Just like in training, it's not just a matter of how much (how much weight to lift, how many kilometers to run, how many strokes before breathing, etc.), but it's also and above all a matter of what (what type of load I provide to my muscles, what intensity of beats I demand from my heart, what pace I can maintain, and so on).

Four-time CrossFit Games champion Rich Froning Jr. summed it up effectively: "*It's not just about how many calories you eat, but what calories you eat.*" It is scientifically proven that the nutrients you consume affect your athletic performance.

To understand it better, imagine your body as an extraordinarily complex machine. This machine requires high-quality fuel to perform at its peak: this fuel comes from your diet. Let's start with the basics.

Carbohydrates

Carbohydrates are the premium fuel component that powers your body: sports that require endurance, such as long-distance running or cycling, heavily rely on carbohydrates to maintain steady energy. During exercise, your body converts carbohydrates into glucose, which is used to produce energy. Without an adequate source of carbohydrates, your performance can decline rapidly. A practical example is a professional cyclist preparing for a race: his pre-race meal will be rich in complex carbohydrates like whole wheat pasta or rice, a tank of energy. These carbohydrates are processed and stored in muscles and the liver as glycogen, ready to be converted into energy when needed.

Proteins

Proteins are essential for muscle repair and growth. During anaerobic exercise, such as weightlifting or high-intensity training, muscles undergo micro-injuries. These micro-injuries are a natural part of the muscle-building process. To repair and rebuild damaged muscle tissues, the body requires an adequate amount of protein. Proteins are also essential for muscle growth. After a workout, the body activates the protein synthesis process to build new muscle tissues. Providing an adequate amount of high-quality proteins (containing all or most essential amino acids) through the diet is crucial to support this muscle growth process. An athlete engaging in intense anaerobic training will need to provide his body with high-quality proteins to aid in the repair of damaged muscles and the building of new muscle tissues.

Fats

Fats are not the enemy; on the contrary, they play a crucial role in providing energy and supporting your nervous system. Healthy fats, such as those found in olive oil and avocado, play a fundamental role in supporting the nervous system and emotional balance. They are involved in the formation of cell membranes and the production of hormones. An athlete who needs to maintain a clear and focused mind during a race needs omega-3 fats to optimize his brain function. Conversely, a deficiency in these essential fats can compromise the ability to make quick decisions.

Vitamins and Minerals

Vitamins and minerals are nutrients with specific roles ranging from energy production to blood clotting. Without them, your body cannot perform vital tasks. A prominent example is vitamin C, known for its role in supporting the immune system. Athletes, often subjected to high physical stress, can greatly benefit from an adequate intake of this vitamin.

All of this is well-known and widely considered: it is a common perception that the food you put into your body directly affects how much you enjoy your life and how far you can push your performance. A good gin and tonic, as refreshing and satisfying as it may be, is unlikely to provide you with the strength to run a half marathon, just as a steaming plate of plain pasta is unlikely to provide effective post-workout recovery on its own.

Okay, we've made enough preamble; let's delve deeper into the matter. One thing is already known: there is no definitive mix of nutrients, no legendary secret blend that suits everyone and infallibly helps you achieve better results. Starting from this essential concept and with general health as the primary goal, in the next chapters, I will introduce you to the concept of superfoods and, above all, consider one by one some foods that, without excessive effort, you can put on your plate every day and expect them to make you feel and perform better due to their specific properties.

I am not a doctor, nor do I want to replace those who work in scientific fields by training and vocation. I simply enjoy amateur but intense sports (from cycling to running, swimming to weightlifting) and feeling good about myself. That's why I felt the need to delve into the various contents scattered in numerous books and research, and explore analytically - but also understandably - how the wealth of nutrients contained in some "superfoods" can become an ally in reaching your full potential.

What you will find in this book: first of all, an analysis of the main (and lesser-known) superfoods, in terms of macronutrients and other nutrients they can provide. You will then find some functions or objectives that superfoods can contribute to, and you will also understand how to introduce them into your daily diet with some very easy recipes and a simplified shopping list based on your real needs. What you won't find in this book: you won't find a specific diet for you, a ready-made routine, for the simple reason that it would not be correct to tell you how much and what to consume without knowing you thoroughly. However, the weekly menu and recipes can be an excellent foundation to help you build your personalized diet.

I hope that by the end of this book, you too will be able to easily create your strategy, your training... dietary routine.

Let's begin.

2.

THE FUNDAMENTALS
OF SUPERFOODS

Anyone who has set foot in a natural or organic food store or delved into the intricacies of nutrition in recent years is likely to have come across superfoods.

These almost mythical foods are often praised as true heroes of the diet, but what are they exactly? How much substance is there in this proposition that has a strong taste of marketing?

Let's start from the beginning. The term "superfood" was coined to describe nutrient-dense foods that potentially offer various health benefits more immediately. It should be said right away: "superfood" is not an officially recognized scientific term, nor is it a defined list of foods, but rather an expression used to distinguish and market specific foods. All marketing and no science? Not exactly.

While there is no standardized definition, various scientific studies recognize the unique properties of some foods that we could describe as "nutrient-dense" or better yet, functional foods.

Many of the plants and foods for which we now recognize specific functions have, in fact, been used for centuries in various cultures around the world.

The main reason superfoods have gained popularity over the centuries is their ability to contribute to specific functions necessary for the health and physical performance of those who consume them. Take, for example, goji berries: used in traditional Chinese medicine for thousands of years for their antioxidant and anti-inflammatory properties. Or quinoa: a grain native to the Andes considered a sacred food by the Incas and used to promote physical and mental endurance. These are just two quick examples.

By drawing from different cultures and scientific research, we are now able to identify foods globally recognized for their superior nutritional characteristics.

Superfoods are often associated with better digestion, a stronger immune system, and increased energy. It is therefore not surprising that they have become an integral part of many diets, including those of athletes.

Considering superfoods as essential foods specifically for sports can be more broadly linked to their nutrient density, i.e., the richness of nutrients they contain. Athletes often require a higher calorie intake and a greater quantity of essential nutrients to support their energy and muscle needs.

Some functional, unprocessed foods, such as walnuts (rich in healthy fats and protein), conveniently provide many crucial and easily assimilated nutrients.

I will dedicate a separate section to some foods, known to athletes, that could be assimilated to superfoods but are not because they do not contain a sufficiently wide range of nutrients. We are talking, for example, about bananas or eggs.

What interests us here is to first delve into the characteristics of individual superfoods and then understand how their integration into our diet can help us achieve our goal: performing better.

Now it is clearer: the definition of superfood is a synthesis, a simplification of the concepts just discussed. The practical reason behind this denomination remains the need to distinguish some foods from others. And that is precisely where its effectiveness lies: in quickly allowing us to perceive some foods as potentially better than others in promoting well-being and performance.

In conclusion, the vaguely consumeristic narrative that accompanies "modern" foods defined as superfoods is rooted in millennial cultural traditions, supported by a growing body of scientific research that proves, beyond empirical subjective perception, the objectively positive impact on human health over time.

Now, let's discover together why some foods deserve more attention than others and should never be missing from our sports nutrition.

3.

WELL-KNOWN SUPERFOODS

In the previous chapter, we clarified the common concepts that unite superfoods. Now, let's take a closer look at some of the most well-known ones and delve deeper into their typical characteristics. You'll notice that we're not only talking about fruits... inside this chapter, you'll find a "bonus" superfood, to be consumed in moderation ;)

[BLUEBERRIES]

Scientific Name: The genus of blueberries is Vaccinium, and it includes various species, such as Vaccinium myrtillus (wild blueberries), Vaccinium corymbosum (American blueberries or blueberries), Vaccinium uliginosum (bog blueberries), and many others.

Geographical Growing Areas: Blueberries are primarily cultivated in temperate and cold regions of the world. They are widespread in North America, Europe, Canada, and parts of Asia. Some varieties of blueberries grow spontaneously in forests and mountainous areas.

Consumption and Cultures: Blueberries are consumed worldwide and are popular in many cultures. In North America, blueberries are often used to make desserts, cakes, jams, and juices. In Europe, especially in Scandinavia, wild blueberries are a common element of traditional cuisine and are often used to prepare sauces for meat or desserts. Blueberries are also known in many Asian cuisines, where they are used in sweet and savory dishes.

Harvest Season: The blueberry harvest season can vary depending on the species and geographical region. In general, blueberries ripen during the summer and fall. For example, American blueberries (Vaccinium corymbosum) are often ready for harvest between June and August in the United States. Wild blueberries (Vaccinium myrtillus) grow in European forests and are generally ready for harvest between July and September.

Varieties: There are numerous varieties of blueberries, each with its own flavor characteristics and adaptability to different climatic conditions. For example, among American blueberry varieties, there are "Bluecrop," "Jersey," "Elliot," and many others. Wild blueberry varieties can also vary depending on the region, but they are generally smaller and darker than American blueberries.

Ways of Consumption: Blueberries can be consumed in various forms, including fresh, frozen, dried, in powder form, or as juices and jams. They are often added to cereals, yogurt, salads, and smoothies. They are a common ingredient in desserts, cakes, muffins, and pancakes.

Average Composition per 100g of Fresh Blueberries:
- Calories: about 43 kcal
- Carbohydrates: about 9.7 g
- Sugars: about 4.9 g
- Fiber: about 2.4 g
- Protein: about 0.7 g
- Fat: about 0.4 g
- Other Elements (in variable amounts): vitamin C and vitamin K, antioxidants such as anthocyanins, quercetin, and resveratrol.

Superfood Characteristics: Blueberries, with their intense blue color and sweet-tart flavor, are a concentrated source of antioxidants, contributing to their health benefits, including support for cognitive function, cardiovascular protection, and anti-inflammatory effects. Among the antioxidants found in blueberries are anthocyanins, which can help protect cells from free radical damage, reduce inflammation, and improve overall health. Scientific studies have suggested that blueberries may also play a role in brain and memory protection, making them a valuable ally in preventing neurodegenerative diseases. Blueberries are also a good source of essential vitamins and minerals, in addition to being relatively low in calories and fats, making them a popular superfood for a balanced diet.

In a broader context, all types of berries (from strawberries to raspberries, currants, blackberries, and many others) are often considered superfoods due to their richness in antioxidants, primarily anthocyanins, vitamins, and fiber.

[KALE]

Scientific Name: Brassica oleracea var. acephala, part of the Brassicaceae family, the same family to which cauliflower, broccoli, and cabbage belong.

Geographical Growing Areas: Kale is originally from the Mediterranean region but is now cultivated worldwide. Major growing regions include Italy, Spain, the United States (especially California), the United Kingdom, and New Zealand.

Consumption and Cultures: Kale is a key ingredient in Italian cuisine, particularly in Tuscany, where it is used in traditional dishes like "Ribollita." In addition to Italy, kale has become popular in other international cuisines, including American, where it is often used in soups and salads.

Harvest Season: The best season for kale harvest is in the fall and winter. Cooler temperatures make the leaves tender and sweeter in taste.

Varieties: The most common variety of kale has dark green, curly leaves. There are also smooth or purple-leaved varieties, but Tuscan kale is the most well-known.

Ways of Consumption: Kale is consumed in various ways: fresh, boiled, baked, or sautéed. It is a versatile ingredient that can be added to a variety of dishes, including soups, pasta, salads, and side dishes. It can also be dried and powdered for use as a seasoning or supplement.

Average Composition per 100g of Fresh Kale:
  - Calories: about 33 kcal
  - Carbohydrates: about 6.7 g
  - Sugars: about 0.9 g
  - Protein: about 2.9 g
  - Fat: about 0.6 g
  - Fiber: about 3.6 g

- Vitamin A: about 474% Recommended Daily Intake (RDI)
- Vitamin K: about 681% RDI
- Vitamin C: about 89% RDI
- Other Elements (in variable amounts): calcium, iron, potassium.

Superfood Characteristics: Kale is considered a superfood thanks to its exceptional nutrient density. It is rich in vitamins A, K, and C, which are essential for eye health, bone health, and the immune system. The chemical composition of kale makes it particularly beneficial for a balanced diet and overall health.

Vitamins A and K are particularly abundant in kale and play crucial roles in disease prevention, blood clotting, and bone health. Vitamin C, on the other hand, is a powerful antioxidant that helps combat oxidative stress. Kale is also a good source of calcium, important for bone health, and potassium, essential for muscle and heart function. Its combination of essential nutrients and antioxidants makes it a valuable element for a balanced diet and the promotion of overall health.

[QUINOA]

Scientific Name: Chenopodium quinoa, quinoa belongs to the Amaranthaceae family, the same family as Swiss chard or spinach.

Geographical Cultivation Zones: Quinoa is native to the Andes in South America, but today it is grown in many parts of the world. The major producing countries include Peru, Bolivia, Ecuador, Colombia, and the United States.

Consumption and Cultures Using It: Quinoa has been a staple in Andean cultures for centuries, used in various traditional dishes like "chuño" and "quinotto." In recent years, quinoa has gained popularity worldwide as a healthy and versatile food, widely consumed in many international cuisines.

Harvest Season: Quinoa is generally cultivated during the rainy season and harvested in the autumn.

Varieties: There are several varieties of quinoa, including white, red, and black quinoa. Each variety has a slightly different flavor and can be used similarly in cooking.

Methods of Consumption: Quinoa is typically sold in seed form and must be cooked before consumption (quick-cooking quinoa is ready in 10 minutes in boiling water). It can be cooked like rice and used as a base for salads, soups, side dishes, or as a cereal alternative for breakfast. Quinoa is also available in the form of flour and flakes and is used to make baked goods like bread and cookies.

Average Composition per 100g of Quinoa:
- Calories: about 360 kcal
- Carbohydrates: about 64 g
- Sugars: about 3.5 g
- Protein: about 12 g
- Fat: about 5.8 g
- Fiber: about 6.8 g
- Vitamin B6: about 9% RDI
- Folate: about 19% RDI
- Magnesium: about 16% RDI
- Other Elements (in varying amounts): phosphorus, iron, zinc.

Superfood Characteristics: Quinoa is considered a superfood due to its exceptional nutritional composition. It is one of the few plant sources that provide complete proteins, containing all the essential amino acids necessary for the human body. This makes it particularly valuable for vegetarians and vegans.

Additionally, quinoa is a good source of dietary fiber, B vitamins, magnesium, and phosphorus. It also contains antioxidants like quercetin and kaempferol. Quinoa is gluten-free, making it suitable for people with celiac disease or gluten sensitivity.

Its combination of complete proteins, complex carbohydrates, fiber, and micronutrients makes it an ideal food for sustained energy, muscle growth, and overall health. It is also highly versatile in the kitchen, making it easy to incorporate into a variety of healthy dishes. Studies suggest that regular consumption of quinoa can contribute to weight control and reduce the risk of certain chronic diseases.

[CHIA SEEDS]

Scientific Name: Chia seeds, known as Salvia hispanica, belong to the Lamiaceae family, which also includes other aromatic plants like mint and basil.

Geographical Cultivation Zones: Originally cultivated in Mexico and surrounding regions, chia seeds are now grown in many parts of the world, including the United States, Argentina, Australia, and Europe.

Consumption and Cultures Using Them: Chia seeds were a significant part of the diets of ancient Aztec and Maya civilizations. Today, they are consumed worldwide for their health benefits. They are often used in smoothies, yogurt, cereals, salads, and can also serve as a natural thickening agent in vegan recipes, replacing eggs in desserts, for example.

Harvest Season: The harvest season for chia seeds can vary depending on the region in which they are grown. Typically, harvesting occurs between March and April.

Varieties: Chia seed varieties may differ slightly in color, with some producing black seeds and others white or gray seeds. However, the nutritional differences between varieties are minimal.

Methods of Consumption: Chia seeds are generally consumed raw. They can be added to beverages, foods, or used to create a gel-like consistency when mixed with liquids. This feature makes them useful in many recipes, such as puddings or desserts.

Average Composition per 100g of Chia Seeds:
- Calories: about 486 kcal
- Carbohydrates: about 42 g
- Sugars: about 0 g
- Protein: about 16.5 g
- Fat: about 30.7 g (primarily polyunsaturated fatty acids, including alpha-linolenic omega-3 fatty acid)
- Fiber: about 34.4 g
- Vitamin B1 (Thiamine): about 0.6 mg, approximately 43% Recommended Daily Intake (RDI)
- Vitamin B3 (Niacin): about 8.8 mg, about 55% RDI
- Calcium: about 631 mg, about 63% RDI
- Phosphorus: about 860 mg, about 86% RDI
- Magnesium: about 335 mg, about 84% RDI

Superfood Characteristics: Chia seeds are considered a superfood due to their exceptional nutritional density (a common characteristic among many superfoods!). Small but powerful, they are one of the richest plant sources of omega-3 fatty acids, which are beneficial for heart and brain health as well as having anti-inflammatory properties. Additionally, they are a good source of protein, fiber, calcium, magnesium, and other essential nutrients.

Their high calcium content makes them suitable for supporting bone health, while their high fiber content can promote good digestion and help maintain stable blood sugar levels.

Chia seeds' ability to absorb water and form a gel makes them useful for enhancing satiety and regulating blood sugar levels. This makes them a valuable addition to weight loss diets and diabetes management. In general, chia seeds are versatile and easy to incorporate into daily diets, making them a popular choice for those looking to improve their health through nutrition.

[AVOCADO]

Scientific Name: Avocado belongs to the Lauraceae family and is scientifically known as Persea americana. Other plants in the same family include cinnamon and laurel.

Geographical Cultivation Zones: Avocado is native to Central and South America but is grown worldwide in tropical and subtropical regions. Some major producing areas include Mexico, the United States (California and Florida), Brazil, Indonesia, and many Latin American countries.

Consumption and Cultures Using It: Avocado is a highly popular food worldwide, but it is particularly consumed in Mexico, where it is a fundamental ingredient in guacamole. It is widely used in cuisine as a condiment, often spread on toast or used in salads and Mexican dishes. Its popularity is continually growing in many other cultures, thanks to its health benefits.

Harvest Season: The avocado harvest season varies depending on the region but generally spans from spring to autumn. In some areas, avocados are available year-round due to the diversity of avocado varieties and imports.

Varieties: Numerous avocado varieties exist, including Hass, Fuerte, Bacon, Pinkerton, and many others. The Hass variety is the most common and is appreciated for its rough skin and buttery flavor.

Methods of Consumption: Avocado is mainly consumed fresh. It is cut in half, the pit is removed, and the flesh is often scooped out with a spoon. It can be added to salads, spread on toast, used to prepare guacamole, or as a condiment for many other dishes. Additionally, avocado-based products like avocado oil and even avocado ice cream can be found.

Average Composition per 100g of Fresh Avocado:
- Calories: about 160 kcal
- Carbohydrates: about 8.53 g
- Sugars: about 0.2 g
- Protein: about 2 g
- Fat: about 14.66 g (mainly monounsaturated fats, known for their heart-healthy benefits)
- Fiber: about 6.7 g
- Vitamin K: about 21 mg, about 26% RDI
- Vitamin C: about 10 mg, about 17% RDI
- Vitamin E: about 2.07 mg, about 14% RDI
- Vitamin B6: about 0.257 mg, about 20% RDI
- Other Elements (in varying amounts): folate, potassium.

Superfood Characteristics: Avocado is considered a superfood primarily due to its richness in monounsaturated fats, including oleic acid, which is known for its positive effects on heart health and cholesterol levels. Additionally, it is a good source of dietary fiber, vitamins (such as vitamin K, vitamin C, vitamin E, vitamin B6, and folate), and minerals like potassium, which plays a key role in maintaining electrolyte balance and regulating blood pressure. Its content of antioxidants, including lutein, can contribute to eye health.

Avocado is known for its rich, buttery flavor, making it a delicious addition to many culinary preparations. Its versatility in the kitchen, combined with its health benefits, makes it a cherished food for those seeking a balanced diet and those looking to harness superfoods to enhance their well-being.

[WILD SALMON]

Scientific Name: Wild salmon belongs to the Salmonidae family and is part of the Oncorhynchus genus. Other members of the Salmonidae family include trout and herring.

Geographical Habitat: Wild salmon are known to inhabit various areas in the northern hemisphere, including the northeastern Pacific and the northwestern Atlantic.

Consumption and Cultures Using It: Wild salmon has been a crucial food source for coastal communities in many parts of the world, including Alaska, Canada, Norway, Scotland, and many other northern regions. It is an integral part of many local cuisines and is widely appreciated for its rich flavor and tender texture.

Fishing Season: The wild salmon fishing season varies depending on the region. In some areas, fishing can be seasonal, while in others, salmon can be caught year-round due to the presence of different species and fisheries management.

Varieties: Several species of wild salmon exist, including king salmon (chinook), pink salmon, sockeye salmon, and others. Each of these species has a slightly different taste and texture.

Methods of Consumption: Wild salmon can be consumed fresh, smoked, canned, or frozen. It is often grilled, baked, or prepared as sushi or sashimi. Salmon oil, extracted from the fatty tissues of the fish, is also used as a dietary supplement.

Average Composition per 100g of Fresh Wild Salmon:

- Calories: about 206 kcal
- Protein: about 22 g
- Fat: about 13 g (including omega-3 fatty acids)
- Carbohydrates: 0 g
- Sugars: 0 g
- Fiber: 0 g
- Vitamin D: about 570 IU (International Units), about 122% Recommended Daily Intake (RDI)
- Vitamin B12: about 5.8 mcg, about 240% RDI
- Vitamin B6: about 0.5 mg, about 25% RDI
- Selenium: about 31.5 mcg, about 57% RDI

Superfood Characteristics: Wild salmon is considered a superfood due to its exceptional concentration of high-quality protein, omega-3 fatty acids (particularly eicosapentaenoic acid, EPA, and docosahexaenoic acid, DHA), vitamin D, vitamin B12, and selenium.

The omega-3 fatty acids found in wild salmon are known for their beneficial effects on heart health, reducing the risk of cardiovascular diseases. Vitamin D in salmon is essential for bone health and the immune system. Vitamin B12 is crucial for the formation of blood cells and the functioning of the nervous system.

Selenium is a potent antioxidant that helps protect cells from oxidative damage.

Wild or Farmed? The consumption of wild salmon is often preferable to farmed salmon for several reasons, including:

- Superior Nutritional Composition: Wild salmon tends to have a superior nutritional composition compared to farmed salmon. Wild salmon grow in natural habitats where they feed on a diverse diet, including small fish, crustaceans, and marine algae. This kind of diet contributes to higher levels of omega-3 fatty acids, high-quality proteins, and vitamins in the fish's meat.
- Lower Contaminant Levels: Wild salmon tends to accumulate fewer environmental contaminants than farmed salmon. Since farmed salmon are often kept in confined spaces, they can be more susceptible to accumulating pesticides, antibiotics, and heavy metals present in water and the food they receive.
- Environmental Sustainability: Wild salmon fishing can be managed sustainably, helping to preserve marine ecosystems and maintain stable salmon populations. On the other hand, large-scale farmed

salmon production can lead to environmental issues like water pollution and the spread of diseases among farmed fish.

- Taste and Texture: Many people prefer the taste and texture of wild salmon, which is often described as more robust and distinctive compared to farmed salmon.

[ACAI]

Scientific Name: The scientific name of açaí is Euterpe oleracea, and it belongs to the palm family (Arecaceae).

Geographical Cultivation Zones: Açaí is native to tropical regions of Central and South America, particularly in Brazil, Colombia, Venezuela, and some parts of the Caribbean islands. It is primarily cultivated in these regions, but due to its growing popularity, açaí cultivation has spread to other parts of the world, including the United States.

Consumption and Cultures Using It: Açaí is a traditional food in Brazilian Amazon cultures, where it has been consumed for centuries. In recent decades, it has gained international popularity as a superfood, mainly due to its antioxidant properties. Today, açaí is widely used worldwide, especially in the preparation of smoothies, açaí bowls, and dietary supplements.

Harvest Season: Açaí is generally harvested year-round in the tropical regions where it grows. The fruits mature during the rainy season and can be harvested when they reach the right level of ripeness.

Varieties: There are several varieties of açaí, but the most well-known are black açaí (Euterpe oleracea) and white açaí (Euterpe edulis). Black açaí is the most common and widespread variety.

Methods of Consumption: Açaí is commonly consumed in the form of a puree or pulp. It can be served as a dessert or snack, often topped with fresh fruit, granola, shredded coconut, or honey. In many cases, it is frozen or freeze-dried to preserve freshness and facilitate distribution.

Average Composition per 100g of Fresh Açaí:
- Calories: About 70-90 kcal
- Carbohydrates: About 4-5 g
- Sugars: About 2 g

- Protein: About 1-2 g
- Fat: About 5-6 g
- Fiber: About 2-3 g
- Other Elements (in varying amounts): anthocyanins, vitamin A, vitamin C, calcium, and potassium.

Superfood Characteristics: Açaí is often considered a superfood due to its high content of antioxidants, which can help combat oxidative stress in the body. The anthocyanins present in açaí have been associated with various health benefits, including heart protection and reduced inflammation. Additionally, açaí is a good source of healthy monounsaturated fats, which can support heart health, and fiber, which promotes digestion and satiety. However, it's important to note that to maximize the benefits, it's preferable to consume açaí in its natural form rather than in highly processed products with added sugars.

[SPIRULINA]

Scientific Name: Spirulina is the common name for various species, including Arthrospira platensis and Arthrospira maxima. These organisms are classified as cyanobacteria but are commonly known as blue-green algae.

Geographical Cultivation Zones: Spirulina grows in many parts of the world but is often cultivated in areas with freshwater or brackish water, such as lakes, ponds, and controlled tanks. Countries like India, China, Mexico, and the United States are among the major spirulina producers.

Consumption and Cultures Using It: Spirulina is consumed worldwide and is often used as a dietary supplement due to its nutritional density. It is particularly popular among vegetarians and vegans for its high protein content. In some cultures, spirulina is a traditional food and is consumed as part of the daily diet.

Harvest Season: Spirulina can be cultivated in controlled environments year-round, meaning it is not tied to a specific harvesting season.

Varieties: The two main species of spirulina are Arthrospira platensis and Arthrospira maxima, but there are other less common species. The difference between these two species mainly concerns their nutritional composition, but both are generally considered suitable for human consumption.

Methods of Consumption: Spirulina is usually sold in the form of powder or tablets. Spirulina powder can be added to smoothies, juices, yogurt, cereals, or beverages as a dietary supplement. Spirulina tablets are easy to consume as a dietary supplement.

Average Composition per 100g of Fresh Spirulina:
- Calories: About 290 kcal
- Carbohydrates: About 23-26 g
- Sugars: About 3-4 g
- Protein: About 57-63 g
- Fat: About 5-7 g
- Fiber: About 3-4 g
- Other Elements (in varying amounts): chlorophyll, vitamin B12, iron, and calcium.

Superfood Characteristics: Spirulina is often considered a superfood due to its high protein content and the presence of essential nutrients such as iron and vitamin B12. It is known for its potential to boost energy and support overall health. Spirulina also contains antioxidants, which can help combat free radicals in the body. However, it's important to note that spirulina can vary in its nutritional composition depending on sources and cultivation methods, so it's important to purchase high-quality, uncontaminated products from reliable sources.

[WALNUTS]

Scientific Name: Walnuts belong to the Juglandaceae family, and their scientific name is Juglans regia.

Geographical Cultivation Zones: Walnuts are cultivated in many parts of the world, with some of the major producing regions including the United States (particularly California), China, Iran, and Turkey. The walnut is native to Central Asia but has been cultivated in many temperate regions.

Consumption and Cultures Using It: Walnuts are consumed worldwide and are a common component of many cuisines. They are used in salads, desserts, bread, and as snacks. They are appreciated for their rich, crunchy flavor and their high content of healthy fats.

Harvest Season: Walnuts are typically harvested in the fall when the shells have hardened, and their contents are mature.

Varieties: There are several varieties of walnuts, including common walnuts (Juglans regia), black walnuts (Juglans nigra), pecans (Carya illinoinensis), and many others.

Methods of Consumption: Walnuts are primarily consumed as a snack but are also a popular ingredient in many dishes. They can be eaten raw or roasted and are often used in both sweet and savory recipes. Chopped walnuts are used to enhance salads and main dishes.

Average Composition per 100g of Walnuts:
- Calories: About 654 kcal
- Carbohydrates: About 13.7 g
- Sugars: About 2.6 g
- Protein: About 15.2 g
- Fat: About 65.2 g
- Fiber: About 6.7 g
- Other Elements (in varying amounts): monounsaturated and polyunsaturated fatty acids,

omega-3 fatty acids, vitamin E, magnesium, and manganese.

Superfood Characteristics: Walnuts are considered a superfood due to their unique nutritional profile. They are exceptionally rich in healthy fats, but they also provide protein, fiber, and antioxidants. However, it's important to consume them in moderation as they are quite calorie-dense. Eating a handful of walnuts per day can help improve cholesterol levels and promote satiety.

[FLAXSEEDS]

Scientific Name: Linum usitatissimum, flax belongs to the Linaceae family.

Geographical Cultivation Zones: Flaxseeds are cultivated in various parts of the world, including Canada, the United States, Russia, China, and India. Canada is one of the world's leading producers of flaxseeds.

Consumption and Cultures Using It: Flaxseeds are consumed in many cultures worldwide. They are often used as a dietary supplement or added to various dishes like cereals, yogurt, salads, and smoothies. They are particularly popular among those following vegetarian or vegan diets as a source of omega-3 fatty acids.

Harvest Season: Flaxseeds are generally sown in the spring and harvested in the summer. The harvesting season can vary depending on climate conditions and the variety of flax.

Varieties: There are several varieties of flaxseeds, but the two main ones are golden flaxseed and brown flaxseed. Both varieties are rich in beneficial nutrients.

Methods of Consumption: Flaxseeds can be consumed whole or ground. They are often ground to make the nutrients more available to the body. They can be added to various dishes such as cereals, yogurt, smoothies, bread, or salads. They can also be used as an egg substitute in some vegan recipes by mixing ground flaxseeds with water.

Average Composition per 100g of Flaxseeds:
- Calories: About 534 kcal
- Carbohydrates: About 28.9 g
- Sugars: About 1.6 g

- Protein: About 18.3 g
- Fat: About 42.2 g
- Fiber: About 27.3 g
- Other Elements (in varying amounts): alpha-linolenic acid (ALA), B-group vitamins (especially thiamine and folates), magnesium, and manganese.

Superfood Characteristics: Flaxseeds are considered a superfood mainly because of their high content of omega-3 fatty acids (among the best in the plant kingdom). The fiber in flaxseeds can contribute to improved digestive health and blood glucose regulation. Additionally, flaxseeds contain lignans, compounds with potential antioxidant and anti-inflammatory properties.

[DARK CHOCOLATE]

Scientific Name: Cocoa, the main ingredient in dark chocolate, comes from the plant known as Theobroma cacao, which belongs to the Sterculiaceae family.

Geographical Cultivation Zones: Cocoa is primarily cultivated in tropical regions, including West Africa, Latin America, and Southeast Asia. Some of the major cocoa-producing countries include Ivory Coast, Ghana, Indonesia, Ecuador, and Nigeria.

Consumption and Cultures Using It: Chocolate, derived from cocoa, is consumed worldwide and is an important part of the culinary culture in many societies. It is used in various sweet products, including chocolate bars, chocolates, spreads, and hot chocolate beverages.

Harvest Season: The cocoa harvest season can vary by region, but in many areas, harvesting occurs throughout the year, with major and minor harvest periods.

Varieties: There are several varieties of cocoa, each with its own flavor characteristics. Some of the most well-known varieties include criollo, forastero, and trinitario.

Methods of Consumption: Dark chocolate can be consumed in various forms, from bars to chocolate chips or cocoa powder. It can be eaten on its own or added to your desserts and treats.

Average Composition per 100g of Dark Chocolate:
- Calories: About 546 kcal
- Carbohydrates: About 60.5 g

- Sugars: About 47.9 g
- Protein: About 4.9 g
- Fat: About 31.3 g
- Fiber: About 7.1 g
- Other Elements (in varying amounts): iron, magnesium, copper, manganese, niacin, pantothenic acid, flavonoids.

Superfood Characteristics: Yes, good news, even dark chocolate can be considered a superfood. When consumed in moderation, it can offer health benefits due to its rich nutrient content and its antioxidants. In particular, flavonoids are known to support heart health, improve blood circulation, and contribute to lower blood pressure. However, make sure that dark chocolate contains at least 70% cocoa to maximize its benefits and reduce the consumption of added sugars.

[TURMERIC]

Scientific Name: Curcuma longa is part of the Zingiberaceae family, to which ginger also belongs.

Geographical Cultivation Zones: Turmeric is native to the Indian subcontinent but is cultivated in many parts of

Asia, Africa, and even some regions of Latin America. Countries like India, Thailand, Indonesia, and Bangladesh are among the major producers of turmeric.

Consumption and Cultures Using It: Turmeric is a widely used ingredient in many Asian cuisines, especially in Indian cuisine. It is a key component of curry powder and imparts a bright yellow color to dishes. Turmeric is also used as a spice and a natural food colorant. Besides its culinary use, turmeric has traditionally been used in Ayurvedic medicine and other traditional healing practices for its purported health benefits.

Harvest Season: Turmeric is generally harvested during the rainy season, which is when the plant thrives.

Varieties: The most common variety of turmeric is "Curcuma longa," but there are several other varieties, each with slight differences in flavor and chemical composition.

Methods of Consumption: Turmeric is available mainly in the form of fresh root, turmeric powder, and supplements. Fresh turmeric root can be used to prepare curries, soups, and meat or fish dishes. Turmeric powder is a spice used to season and color various dishes. Turmeric supplements are popular for those who want to benefit from its potential healing properties without using it in daily cooking.

Average Composition per 100g of Turmeric Powder:
- Calories: About 354 kcal
- Carbohydrates: About 64.9 g
- Sugars: About 3.2 g
- Protein: About 7.8 g
- Fat: About 9.9 g
- Fiber: About 21 g

Superfood Characteristics: Turmeric is considered a superfood mainly because of its curcumin content, an active compound with potential antioxidant and anti-inflammatory properties. Turmeric has been studied for its role in reducing inflammation, protecting cells from free radical damage, and supporting joint health. Turmeric is also used to alleviate digestive issues like nausea, bloating, and diarrhea. However, it's important to note that the human body has difficulty absorbing curcumin, but there are ways to enhance its bioavailability, such as adding black pepper to the diet.

[GREEK YOGURT]

Consumption and Cultures Using It: Greek yogurt consumption is widespread in Greece but is also popular in many other parts of the world, including Western countries. It is appreciated for its creamy texture and rich flavor. Its production is global and involves the fermentation of dairy.

Varieties: There are various varieties of Greek yogurt, with the main variation being the amount of fat and protein in the product.

Methods of Consumption: Greek yogurt is consumed fresh, often on its own or as part of sweet or savory dishes. It is often served with honey and fruits as a dessert or breakfast item. It is also a common ingredient in salads and dressings.

Average Composition per 100g of Greek Yogurt:
- Calories: About 100 kcal
- Carbohydrates: About 3.6 g
- Sugars: About 3.6 g
- Protein: About 10 g
- Fat: About 5 g

- Fiber: Traces
- Other Elements (in varying amounts): probiotics

Superfood Characteristics: Greek yogurt is considered a superfood primarily because it is a good source of protein and calcium, as well as the probiotics naturally present in it. The probiotics in Greek yogurt are live microorganisms, commonly two strains of beneficial bacteria, Lactobacillus bulgaricus and Bifidobacterium lactis. These bacteria work synergistically to promote gut health and support the immune system. Its versatility makes it a useful component for a variety of dishes, making it a nutritious and delicious choice.

[GREEN TEA]

Scientific Name: Green tea is obtained from the leaves of the Camellia sinensis plant.

Geographical Cultivation Zones: Green tea is primarily cultivated in China, Japan, India, and many other regions of Asia, but it is also grown in some other parts of the world.

Consumption and Cultures Using It: Green tea is widely consumed in many Asian cultures, especially in China and Japan, where it is an integral part of culinary tradition and ceremonies. However, its consumption has spread worldwide in recent years due to its health benefits.

Harvest Season: The harvesting of green tea leaves occurs during spring and summer, depending on the varieties and regions.

Varieties: There are many varieties of green tea, each with slightly different taste characteristics. Some of the most well-known varieties include Japanese Sencha green tea, Chinese Dragon Well, Matcha (powdered green tea), and Japanese Gyokuro.

Methods of Consumption: Green tea can be consumed as a hot or cold beverage. It can be prepared simply by steeping tea leaves in hot water or used as an ingredient in a variety of dishes, desserts, and even cocktails. Matcha, for example, is green tea powder used to prepare a thick and creamy beverage.

Average Composition per 100g of Green Tea:

- Calories: About 1-2 kcal
- Carbohydrates: About 0.2-0.4 g
- Sugars: About 0 g
- Protein: About 0.1-0.2 g
- Fat: About 0 g
- Fiber: About 0.2-0.4 g
- Other Elements (in varying amounts): vitamin C, B-group vitamins, fluoride, potassium, and manganese. catechins.

Superfood Characteristics: Green tea is considered a superfood thanks to its rich concentration of antioxidants, particularly catechins. These compounds have demonstrated health benefits, including the ability to combat free radicals, improve brain function, support weight loss, and promote heart health. Green tea is also associated with a range of other potential health benefits, including a reduced risk of certain chronic diseases and increased metabolism. Its long history of use in traditional Asian medicine is a testament to its reputation as a healthful food.

[SPINACH]

Scientific Name: Spinach belongs to the Chenopodiaceae family and the species Spinacia oleracea.

Geographical Cultivation Zones: Spinach is grown in many regions of the world but is native to Western Asia. It is widely cultivated in Europe, North America, and other parts of Asia.

Consumption and Cultures Using It: Spinach is consumed worldwide and is used in various culinary preparations, including salads, side dishes, soups, fillings, and much more. It is particularly popular in Italian, French, and Mediterranean cuisines.

Harvest Season: Spinach is usually harvested during the spring and fall, but it can be grown and harvested in greenhouses throughout the year.

Varieties: There are several varieties of spinach, including smooth-leaf and curly-leaf types. Some varieties are known to be more tender and flavorful, while others are suitable for specific purposes, such as baby spinach production.

Methods of Consumption: Spinach can be consumed fresh in salads, cooked as a side dish, or used in green smoothies or juices for a healthier option. Additionally, it is available as an ingredient in food products such as pasta, bread, and sauces.

Average Composition per 100g of Fresh Spinach:
- Calories: About 23 kcal
- Carbohydrates: About 3.6 g
- Sugars: About 0.4 g
- Protein: About 2.9 g
- Fat: About 0.4 g
- Fiber: About 2.2 g
- Vitamin A: About 188% of the recommended daily intake (RDI)
- Vitamin C: About 47% of RDI
- Vitamin K: About 604% of RDI
- Other Elements (in varying amounts): iron, calcium, potassium.

Superfood Characteristics: Spinach is considered a superfood due to its exceptional density of vitamins, especially vitamin K, vitamin A, and vitamin C, which play crucial roles in bone health, vision, and immunity. Spinach is also a significant source of iron, which is essential for oxygen transport in the body. Furthermore, it is a good source of antioxidants like lutein and zeaxanthin, which can contribute to protecting the eyes from age-related damage. Its fiber contributes to digestive health and may help regulate body weight. Spinach is a highly versatile food that can be easily incorporated into a healthy diet.

These functional foods are just the beginning of our journey into the world of optimal nutrition. Before delving into specific functions achievable through these foods, in the next chapter, we will explore other, less-known superfoods.

4.

LESS COMMON SUPERFOODS

In our journey of exploring superfoods, it's important to also examine those that are less known but equally powerful.

[BAOBAB]

Scientific Name: Baobab is scientifically known as Adansonia and belongs to the Malvaceae family.

Geographical Cultivation Zones: Baobab grows in various parts of Africa, particularly in sub-Saharan Africa regions. It is common in countries such as Senegal, Mali, South Africa, Madagascar, and many others.

Consumption and Cultures Using It: Baobab has been an integral part of traditional cuisine in many African cultures for centuries. Various parts of the tree, including the fruit, leaves, and bark, are used as food and a source of water. In Africa, baobab is known as the "tree of life" due to its nutritional significance.

Harvest Season: Baobab fruit ripens during the rainy season, which may vary from one region to another but generally occurs during the African summer.

Varieties: There are several baobab species, but Adansonia digitata is the most commonly cultivated species for food purposes.

Methods of Consumption: Baobab fruit is known for its dry powder, which can be obtained by grinding dried fruit pulp. This powder is highly versatile and can be used in beverages, smoothies, baked goods, yogurt, and more. It is known for its tangy and slightly sweet flavor.

Average Composition per 100g of Baobab Powder:
- Calories: About 330 kcal
- Carbohydrates: About 80 g
- Sugars: About 30 g
- Protein: About 3 g
- Fat: About 0.2 g
- Fiber: About 44 g
- Vitamin C: About 275% of the Recommended Daily Intake (RDI)
- Other Elements (in varying amounts): iron, calcium, potassium, vitamin B6, flavonoids, and polyphenols.

Superfood Characteristics: Baobab is considered a superfood, particularly due to its incredible amount of vitamin C and high fiber content. Additionally, baobab is rich in antioxidants.

[MACA]

Scientific Name: Maca is known as Lepidium meyenii and belongs to the Brassicaceae family.

Geographical Cultivation Zones: Maca, a relative of cabbage and broccoli, is native to the Andes of Peru and is primarily cultivated in the mountainous regions of this country, including the highlands of the central and southern Andes. Besides Peru, it is also grown in other parts of the world, but its main production remains concentrated in Peru.

Consumption and Cultures Using It: Maca has been an important part of the traditional Peruvian diet and medicine for centuries. It is considered an aphrodisiac and is often consumed to increase energy and stamina. Besides Peru, maca has gained popularity worldwide as a dietary supplement.

Harvest Season: Maca is cultivated and harvested primarily between May and November in the Andean regions of Peru.

Varieties: There are several varieties of maca, each with slight color differences (black, red, and yellow) and nutritional properties. The most common and widely available type is yellow maca.

Methods of Consumption: Maca root is commonly sold in the form of powder or capsules as a dietary supplement. It can also be consumed cooked or dried and used in culinary preparations such as soups, stews, cookies, and beverages.

Average Composition per 100g of Maca Powder:
- Calories: About 325 kcal
- Carbohydrates: About 70 g
- Sugars: About 30 g
- Protein: About 10 g
- Fat: About 1.5 g
- Fiber: About 5 g
- Vitamin C: About 50% of the RDI
- Manganese: About 150% of the RDI
- Other Elements (in varying amounts): iron, calcium, potassium.

Superfood Characteristics: Maca is considered a superfood primarily due to its richness in vitamin C, iron, and manganese. It is also notable for its high copper content, which plays a significant role in energy production and red blood cell formation. Maca is often consumed to support energy, stamina, and overall well-being, and it has been the subject of studies regarding its potential to increase libido and fertility, although further research is needed to confirm these effects.

[KELP]

Scientific Name: The name "kelp" is used for several species of Laminariales, which are brown marine algae.

Geographical Cultivation Zones: Kelp is common in the cold and temperate waters of oceans and is often associated with the rocky shores of the northern Atlantic and northwestern Pacific. It is particularly abundant in coastal regions of East Asia, such as Japan and Korea.

Consumption and Cultures Using It: Kelp has been an important part of traditional diets in many coastal cultures, especially in Asia. It is used to prepare various dishes, including soups, salads, rice dishes, and more. Its extract, sodium alginate, is also used in the food industry as a thickening and gelling agent.

Harvest Season: Kelp can be harvested in different seasons of the year, but it is often collected in spring or autumn when it is more abundant and nutritious.

Varieties: There are several kelp species, including Laminaria japonica (kombu), and Saccharina latissima, each with its own characteristics and culinary uses.

Methods of Consumption: Kelp can be consumed fresh or dried and then rehydrated before use. It is often used as a base for broths and soups, as well as a seasoning in Japanese and Korean cuisine. Additionally, it is processed into dietary supplements in the form of capsules or powder.

Average Composition per 100g of Fresh Kelp:
- Calories: About 43 kcal
- Carbohydrates: About 9.6 g
- Sugars: About 0.6 g
- Protein: About 1.7 g
- Fat: About 0.6 g
- Fiber: About 1.3 g
- Other Elements (in varying amounts): Vitamin K, Iodine, Vitamin B12, calcium, potassium, and magnesium.

Superfood Characteristics: Kelp is considered a superfood mainly due to its extraordinary richness in iodine and vitamin K. Iodine is a mineral essential for thyroid health and metabolic regulation, while vitamin K plays a key role in blood clotting and bone health. However, it is important to consume kelp in moderation as excess iodine can cause thyroid problems.

[SORREL]

Scientific Name: Sorrel is Rumex acetosa and belongs to the Polygonaceae family. In Italy, it is known as Acetosa or Acetosella.

Geographical Cultivation Zones: This plant mainly grows in Europe and Asia but is also found in other parts of the world.

Consumption and Cultures Using It: Sorrel has traditionally been used in cuisine in many cultures, including European and Asian. The fresh leaves have a slightly citrusy flavor and are often used in salads, soups, and fish dishes. In some cultures, sorrel is also used to prepare refreshing beverages or sauces.

Harvest Season: Sorrel is typically harvested in spring and early summer when the leaves are tender and flavorful. It can also be grown in gardens for more constant access to fresh leaves.

Varieties: There are several varieties of sorrel, including "common sorrel" (Rumex acetosa) and "French sorrel" (Rumex scutatus).

Methods of Consumption: Sorrel leaves can be consumed fresh, usually in salads or cold dishes, or they can be cooked and used in soups or sauces. Some people also prefer to use them to make herbal teas or infusions.

Average Composition per 100g of Fresh Sorrel:
- Calories: About 22 kcal
- Carbohydrates: About 4.4 g
- Sugars: About 0.9 g
- Protein: About 1.5 g
- Fat: Trace amounts.
- Fiber: About 2.8 g
- Other Elements (in varying amounts): vitamin C, vitamin A, vitamin K, iron, potassium.

Superfood Characteristics: Sorrel is often considered a superfood for its richness in nutrients, including vitamins and antioxidants like vitamin C and beta-carotene, as well as oxalic acid.

[CAMU CAMU]

Scientific Name: Camu camu belongs to the Myrtaceae family and is scientifically known as Myrciaria dubia.

Geographical Cultivation Zones: It is primarily cultivated in the Amazon regions, especially in Peru and Brazil, but also in Colombia and Venezuela, where it grows in wet and swampy areas.

Consumption and Cultures Using It: Camu camu fruits are traditionally used by local populations in the Amazon.

Harvest Season: The camu camu harvest season varies depending on the region but generally occurs between June and November.

Varieties: Camu camu is generally known in a single variety, but there may be slight variations in vitamin C concentration among plants from different regions.

Methods of Consumption: Camu camu fruits are often processed into powder or juices to facilitate consumption. Camu camu powder is used to enrich beverages, smoothies, yogurt, and more.

Average Composition per 100g of Fresh Camu Camu:
- Calories: About 43 kcal
- Carbohydrates: About 9.8 g
- Sugars: About 2 g
- Protein: About 1 g
- Fat: About 0.2 g
- Fiber: About 1.1 g

Superfood Characteristics: Camu camu is considered a superfood primarily due to its extraordinary concentration of vitamin C, which can exceed 2,000-3,000 milligrams per 100 grams of fresh product, making it one of the richest foods in this vitamin in the world. It is also a source of antioxidants such as flavonoids and carotenoids.

[LUCUMA]

Scientific Name: Lucuma, scientifically known as Pouteria lucuma, is a tree belonging to the Sapotaceae family.

Geographical Cultivation Zones: It is primarily cultivated in the Andean regions of South America, with a particular concentration in Peru, Chile, and Ecuador.

Consumption and Cultures Using It: Lucuma has been used for centuries in cuisine, particularly in Peruvian and Chilean cuisines. Its fruit, with a sweet flavor and a unique texture resembling hard-boiled egg yolk, is used to make sweets, ice creams, smoothies, and other desserts.

Harvest Season: The lucuma harvest season varies, but typically, the fruits ripen between November and April.

Varieties: The "sedo" variety has softer fruit flesh, while the "palo" variety has firmer fruit flesh.

Methods of Consumption: Lucuma is often consumed fresh, but it is also available in the form of dry powder, which is popular as an additive for sweets and smoothies.

Average Composition per 100g of Fresh Lucuma:
- Calories: About 97 kcal
- Carbohydrates: About 23.4 g
- Sugars: About 14.3 g
- Protein: About 2.3 g
- Fat: About 0.5 g
- Fiber: About 2.3 g

Superfood Characteristics: Lucuma is considered a superfood for several reasons. Firstly, it is known for its natural sweet flavor, making it a healthier alternative to sweeten foods compared to refined sugar. Additionally, lucuma is a good source of antioxidants, vitamins, and essential minerals, including vitamin B3, iron, and zinc. Finally, lucuma is appreciated for its versatility in cooking, as its sweet and creamy flavor can be used in a variety of sweet preparations, smoothies, and desserts.

[YACÓN]

Scientific Name: Scientifically known as Smallanthus sonchifolius, yacón is a plant belonging to the Asteraceae family.

Geographical Cultivation Zones: It is native to the South American Andes, with a primary distribution in Peru, Colombia, and Bolivia. It is now cultivated in various parts of the world with suitable climates.

Consumption and Cultures Using It: Yacón is a sweet and crunchy tuber traditionally used in Andean regional cuisines. The root can be consumed fresh but is often eaten dried and sold as a sweet snack.

Harvest Season: Yacón is usually harvested between May and November when the tubers reach maturity.

Varieties: The most common variety is Smallanthus sonchifolius.

Methods of Consumption: Unlike sweet potatoes, it can be consumed fresh, but it is more commonly found in the form of dried slices or cubes, similar to sweet chips.

Average Composition per 100g of Fresh Yacón:
  - Calories: About 33 kcal
  - Carbohydrates: About 8.04 g
  - Sugars: About 6.45 g

- Protein: About 0.82 g
- Fat: About 0.19 g
- Fiber: About 1.6 g

Superfood Characteristics: Yacón is considered a superfood primarily because of its fructooligo-saccharides (FOS) content, which are natural prebiotics. These FOS pass through the digestive tract undigested but provide nourishment for beneficial bacteria in the colon, promoting intestinal health and regularity. Additionally, yacón has a very low glycemic index due to its sugar content, making it a suitable choice for people looking to control blood sugar. Its natural sweetness mainly comes from FOS, which are sweet but do not significantly impact blood sugar levels. Yacón is also a good source of fiber, vitamin C, and antioxidants.

[NATTO]

Scientific Name: Stretching it a bit, it can be said that the scientific name of natto is Glycine max. Let's see why.

Geographical Cultivation Zones: Natto is native to Japan and is widespread throughout the country. It is also produced in other parts of the world but is more popular in Japan.

Consumption and Cultures Using It: Natto is widely consumed in Japan and is an integral part of the Japanese diet. It is often eaten for breakfast but can be consumed at any time of the day.

Harvest Season: Natto is not a plant but a fermented soybean product, so it does not have a specific harvest season. Soybeans are grown and harvested when matured for natto production.

Varieties: Natto is primarily soy-based, but there are regional variations and similar products made from other legumes.

Methods of Consumption: Natto is traditionally consumed as a condiment for rice. It is served with soy sauce, Japanese mustard (karashi), and often with chopped green onions. Its texture is sticky and stringy due to bacterial fermentation.

Average Composition per 100g of Fresh Natto:
  - Calories: About 212 kcal

- Carbohydrates: About 14 g
- Sugars: About 0.3 g
- Protein: About 18 g
- Fat: About 11 g
- Fiber: About 5 g
- Other Elements (in varying amounts): vitamin K2, B vitamins, calcium, iron, potassium, and magnesium.

Superfood Characteristics: Natto is considered a superfood because of its richness in high-quality proteins, fiber, vitamins, and minerals. In particular, the presence of vitamin K2, which can contribute to bone health and calcium metabolism, makes it a valuable food. Additionally, the fermentation process of natto can increase the bioavailability of some nutrients and may have positive effects on intestinal health. However, it should be noted that the taste and texture of natto are not liked by everyone, and it is a food that may require some adaptation for unaccustomed palates.

[SACHA INCHI]

Scientific Name: The scientific name of sacha inchi is Plukenetia volubilis. It belongs to the Euphorbiaceae family and is related to other plants like cassava.

Geographical Cultivation Zones: Sacha inchi is native to the Amazon regions of South America, including Peru, Colombia, Ecuador, and some parts of Brazil. Today, it is also cultivated in other parts of the world, including the United States.

Consumption and Cultures Using It: Sacha inchi has traditionally been used by indigenous populations of the Amazon regions as part of their diet. In recent years, it has become popular worldwide as a superfood due to its nutritional composition.

Harvest Season: The harvesting of sacha inchi capsules generally occurs during the dry season but can vary depending on the region.

Varieties: There are several varieties of sacha inchi, but the most common one has capsules containing oil-rich seeds.

Methods of Consumption: Sacha inchi seeds are typically roasted and consumed as snacks. They can also be used as toppings for salads, yogurt, or cereals, or used to extract oil. Sacha inchi oil is valued for its unique lipid profile.

Average Composition per 100g of Fresh Sacha Inchi:
- Calories: About 500-600 kcal
- Carbohydrates: About 23-27 g
- Sugars: About 1-2 g
- Protein: About 27-30 g
- Fat: About 45-50 g
- Fiber: About 6-8 g
- Other Elements (in varying amounts): vitamin E, vitamin A, magnesium, and calcium.

Superfood Characteristics: Sacha inchi is considered a superfood due to its unique nutritional profile, with a balance of high-quality proteins, abundant healthy fats (omega-3), fiber, and vitamins. In particular, the presence of vitamin K2, which can contribute to bone health and calcium metabolism, makes it a valuable food. Additionally, the fermentation process of natto can increase the bioavailability of some nutrients and may have positive effects on intestinal health.

[AMARANTH]

Scientific Name: Amaranth belongs to the genus Amaranthus and the family Amaranthaceae. Other plants in this family include Swiss chard and quinoa.

Geographical Cultivation Zones: Amaranth is native to tropical regions of the Americas, particularly Central and South America. Today, it is grown in many parts of the world, including Asia, Africa, and Europe.

Consumption and Cultures Using It: Amaranth is an ancient grain consumed for thousands of years by various cultures, including the Aztecs and Incas in the Americas. It is still part of the traditional diet in some regions of India, Africa, and Latin America. In many cultures, amaranth is used to prepare dishes like porridge, soups, side dishes, and even desserts.

Harvest Season: Amaranth can be grown in different seasons depending on the region and climatic conditions.

Varieties: There are many varieties of amaranth, but the most commonly cultivated for food purposes are

Amaranthus cruentus, Amaranthus hypochondriacus, and Amaranthus caudatus.

Methods of Consumption: Amaranth can be consumed in various forms, including seeds, flour, flakes, or as fresh or cooked leaves. The seeds can be used to make cereals, baking flour, or even popcorn. Amaranth leaves, similar to spinach leaves, are used in various culinary preparations, especially in vegetable-based dishes.

Average Composition per 100g of Fresh Amaranth:
- Calories: About 370-380 kcal
- Carbohydrates: About 65-75 g
- Sugars: About 1-2 g
- Protein: About 13-14 g
- Fat: About 5-7 g
- Fiber: About 6-8 g
- Other Elements (in varying amounts): vitamin C, vitamin A, B vitamins (particularly folate and riboflavin), and vitamin K. It is also a good source of minerals like calcium, iron, magnesium, phosphorus, and potassium.

Superfood Characteristics: Amaranth is considered a superfood due to its exceptional nutrient density, particularly its high percentage of complete proteins containing all essential amino acids. It is also a good source of dietary fiber, vitamins, and essential minerals. Amaranth is gluten-free, making it an ideal choice for individuals with gluten intolerance. Its seeds also contain bioactive compounds like squalene, which may have health benefits.

Amaranth is valued for its versatility in the kitchen and its remarkable health benefits, including support for digestion, regulation of blood sugar levels, and immune system support. Amaranth can be used in breakfast cereals, energy bars, or as a cereal substitute in baking bread and desserts.

[FENUGREEK]

Scientific Name: The scientific name of fenugreek is Trigonella foenum-graecum. This plant belongs to the Fabaceae family, which also includes legumes like beans, lentils, and peas.

Geographical Cultivation Zones: Fenugreek is native to South Asia and is widely found in India, Pakistan, Egypt, and other Middle Eastern regions. Today, it is cultivated worldwide, including in some regions of Europe and North America.

Consumption and Cultures Using It: Fenugreek has been traditionally used in cooking and natural medicine in many cultures. It is widely used in Indian and Middle Eastern cuisine, where its leaves and seeds are often added to dishes like curry. It is also used in dietary supplements and herbal teas for its health benefits.

Harvest Season: Fenugreek seeds are usually harvested during the summer, while the leaves can be harvested at various times of the year.

Varieties: There are several varieties of fenugreek, but the most common ones have yellow or brown seeds. The variety can slightly influence the flavor and chemical composition.

Methods of Consumption: Fenugreek is consumed mainly in the form of seeds, fresh or dried leaves, seed powder, capsules, or tea. The seeds are often roasted to enhance their flavor and are used in many culinary preparations.

Average Composition per 100g of Fenugreek:
- Calories: About 323 kcal
- Carbohydrates: About 58 g
- Sugars: About 0 g
- Protein: About 23 g
- Fat: About 6 g
- Fiber: About 25 g
- Other Elements (in varying amounts): B vitamins (especially folate and niacin), vitamin A, vitamin C, and vitamin K. It also contains minerals like iron, potassium, calcium, magnesium, and zinc.

Superfood Characteristics: Fenugreek is considered a superfood due to its numerous beneficial properties. It is known to help regulate blood sugar levels, improve digestion, support heart health, and promote breast milk production in breastfeeding mothers. Additionally, fenugreek seeds contain active compounds like trigonelline and diosgenin, which may have antioxidant and anti-inflammatory effects.

[CAMELINA]

Scientific Name: The scientific name of camelina is Camelina sativa. This plant belongs to the Brassicaceae family, which also includes vegetables like broccoli, cabbage, and radishes.

Geographical Cultivation Zones: Camelina is native to Northern Europe and Western Asia. It is mainly cultivated in countries like Canada, the United States, Russia, and some European countries. Its cultivation is becoming increasingly popular due to its health benefits and versatility.

Consumption and Cultures Using It: Camelina has been traditionally used as food and for medicinal purposes in some European cultures. Today, it is considered a "new" oilseed plant with growing popularity, especially for its oil rich in omega-3 fatty acids.

Harvest Season: Camelina is typically sown in spring and harvested in summer or early autumn, depending on local climate conditions.

Varieties: There are different varieties of camelina, but all are primarily grown for their oil-rich seeds.

Methods of Consumption: The most common part of camelina consumed is its oil, known for its healthy fatty acid profile. Camelina oil is used in cooking to dress salads, vegetables, and various dishes. The seeds can also be consumed directly or added to cereals, yogurt, or smoothies.

Average Composition per 100 ml of Camelina Oil:
- Calories: About 534 kcal
- Carbohydrates: About 16 g
- Sugars: About 0 g
- Protein: About 20 g
- Fat: About 45 g
- Fiber: About 37 g
- Other Elements (in varying amounts): omega-3 and omega-6 fatty acids, vitamin E, B vitamins.

Superfood Characteristics: Camelina oil is considered a superfood primarily due to its concentration of polyunsaturated fatty acids, especially omega-3 fatty acids (such as alpha-linolenic acid) and omega-6. However, it is important to note that it is a delicate oil and can become rancid easily, so it must be stored properly.

Each of these superfoods, whether well-known or less so, can offer you a different set of nutrients. Incorporating them into your diet can contribute to improving your overall well-being and provide you with a variety of essential nutrients.

Now that we've taken a close look at various superfoods, let's discover their main functions and how they can benefit your health.

5.

SUPERFOODS THAT "DIDN'T MAKE THE CUT"

There are some foods that haven't become super, in the sense of being super-dense in various nutrients, like the ones we've just seen.

However, these foods can be considered excellent functional allies in sports nutrition. Let's take a closer look at them: they will come in handy when we think about our weekly shopping and diet.

[PEANUTS]

Key Features Peanuts are rich in proteins, healthy fats, and niacin (vitamin B3). They make an excellent post-workout snack for muscle recovery.

Average composition per 100g of peanuts
- Calories: 567 kcal
- Carbohydrates: 16.1 g
- Sugars: 4.7 g
- Proteins: 25.8 g
- Fats: 49.2 g
- Fiber: 8.5 g
- Other Elements (in varying amounts): niacin (vitamin B3), magnesium.

Benefits for Those Who Exercise Peanuts provide essential proteins for muscle recovery and are a source of healthy fats that can help maintain energy during physical activity.

[OATS]

Key Features Oats are a source of slow-release carbohydrates, soluble fibers, proteins, and B-group vitamins. It's an excellent pre-workout food for providing constant energy.

Average composition per 100g of oats
- Calories: 389 kcal
- Carbohydrates: 66.3 g
- Sugars: 0.8 g
- Proteins: 16.9 g
- Fats: 6.9 g
- Fiber: 10.6 g
- Other Elements (in varying amounts): vitamin B1, vitamin B5, iron, magnesium.

Benefits for Those Who Exercise Oats provide complex carbohydrates that help maintain energy during workouts. The fibers help regulate digestion, and vitamin B contributes to energy metabolism.

[BANANAS]

Key Features Bananas are rich in carbohydrates, especially natural sugars like glucose, fructose, and sucrose. They are also a source of potassium, vitamin C, and vitamin B6.

Average composition per 100g of bananas
- Calories: 89 kcal
- Carbohydrates: 22.8 g
- Sugars: 12.2 g
- Proteins: 1.1 g
- Fats: 0.3 g
- Fiber: 2.6 g
- Other Elements (in varying amounts): vitamin C, vitamin B6, potassium.

Benefits for Those Who Exercise Bananas provide rapidly absorbed carbohydrates, useful for a quick energy boost before or during physical activity. Potassium helps prevent muscle cramps during exercise. The present carbohydrates are also slow-release and provide a steady energy supply.

[WHITE MEATS]

Key Features White meats, such as chicken and turkey, are a source of lean and high-quality proteins. They are essential for muscle building and recovery.

Average composition per 100g of white meats
- Calories vary depending on the cut and preparation but are generally less than 200 kcal per 100 g.
- Carbohydrates: 0 g
- Sugars: 0 g
- Proteins: About 30 g
- Fats: About 2-7 g
- Fiber: 0 g
- Other Elements (in varying amounts): B-group vitamins (B1, B2, B3, B5, B6), selenium.

Benefits for Those Who Exercise White meats provide lean proteins and essential amino acids, contributing to muscle growth and recovery. Selenium plays a role as an antioxidant.

[ALMONDS]

Key Features Almonds are rich in heart-healthy monounsaturated fats, proteins, fiber, vitamin E, and magnesium. They are an excellent snack for sustained energy during physical activity.

Average composition per 100g of almonds
- Calories: 576 kcal
- Carbohydrates: 21.7 g
- Sugars: 4.2 g
- Proteins: 21.2 g
- Fats: 49.9 g
- Fiber: 12.2 g
- Other Elements (in varying amounts): vitamin E, magnesium, calcium.

Benefits for Those Who Exercise Almonds provide healthy fats that can be used as an energy source during exercise. They are also rich in proteins and fiber.

[SWEET POTATOES]

Key Features Sweet potatoes are a source of complex carbohydrates high in starch, fiber, vitamin A (beta-carotene), vitamin C, and potassium. They have a natural sweet taste and a low glycemic index.

Average composition per 100g of sweet potatoes
- Calories: about 86 kcal
- Proteins: about 1.6 g
- Fats: about 0.2 g

- Carbohydrates: about 20 g
- Fiber: about 3 g
- Other Elements (in varying amounts): vitamin A (beta-carotene), vitamin C.

Benefits for Those Who Exercise Sweet potatoes provide slow-release carbohydrates, ideal for sustaining energy during workouts. Vitamins A and C contribute to the immune system and skin health.

[FATTY FISH, E.G., MACKEREL]

Key Features Fatty fish, such as mackerel, are rich in high-quality lean proteins and omega-3 fatty acids, like eicosapentaenoic acid (EPA) and docosahexaenoic acid (DHA), which have anti-inflammatory properties and support cardiovascular health.

Average composition per 100g of mackerel
- Calories: about 205 kcal
- Proteins: about 24 g
- Fats: about 13.4 g
- Carbohydrates: 0 g
- Other Elements (in varying amounts): omega-3 (EPA and DHA), vitamin D.

Benefits for Those Who Exercise Fish provides high-quality proteins for muscle repair, while omega-3s help reduce inflammation, promoting better recovery after exercise. Vitamin D contributes to bone health.

[WHOLE GRAIN RICE]

Key Features Whole grain rice is a source of complex carbohydrates, fiber, B-group vitamins, minerals like magnesium and selenium, and antioxidants.

Composition per 100g of whole grain rice
- Calories: about 130 kcal
- Proteins: about 2.7 g
- Fats: about 0.6 g
- Carbohydrates: about 28.2 g
- Fiber: about 2.8 g
- Other Elements (in varying amounts): vitamin B1, vitamin B3, magnesium.

Benefits for Those Who Exercise Whole grain rice provides carbohydrates for energy, and B-group vitamins contribute to energy metabolism. Fiber supports digestion.

[EXTRA VIRGIN OLIVE OIL]

Key Features Extra virgin olive oil is a source of monounsaturated fats, especially oleic acid, known for its heart health benefits. It also contains antioxidants like vitamin E.

Composition per 100 milliliters of extra virgin olive oil
- Calories: about 884 kcal
- Fats: about 100 g
- Proteins: 0 g
- Carbohydrates: 0 g
- Other Elements (in varying amounts): vitamin E.

Benefits for Those Who Exercise Extra virgin olive oil can be used as a healthy condiment in food preparations. Monounsaturated fatty acids promote cardiovascular health.

[EGGS]

Key Features Eggs are a complete source of proteins and contain all essential amino acids. They are rich in vitamins (B2, B6, B12, D) and minerals (iron, zinc).

Average composition per 100g of eggs
- Calories: About 143 kcal
- Carbohydrates: 1.1 g
- Sugars: 0.6 g
- Proteins: About 13 g
- Fats: About 10.6 g
- Fiber: 0 g
- Other Elements (in varying amounts): vitamin B2, vitamin B6, vitamin B12, vitamin D, iron, zinc.

Benefits for Those Who Exercise Eggs provide high-quality proteins essential for muscle repair. Vitamin D supports bone health.

6.

FUNCTIONS AND OBJECTIVES SUPERFOODS CAN CONTRIBUTE TO

Now we can group the various superfoods we've learned about into specific categories. These are functional foods, particularly suitable for certain purposes.

As mentioned, the physical performance of both professional athletes and amateurs depends not only on the quantity and quality of their training but also, to a significant extent, on a balanced and targeted diet. Superfoods can play a crucial role in enhancing energy, endurance, muscle repair, and many other essential aspects for sports enthusiasts.

SUPERFOODS FOR ENERGY AND ENDURANCE

Energy is the fundamental fuel for any physical activity, and athletes rely on a constant supply of energy to achieve their optimal performance. Do you engage in endurance sports or activities that require a constant energy supply? Let's look at some superfoods that can boost your energy:

QUINOA: Quinoa is a complete grain that offers complex carbohydrates, fiber, and protein. This combination provides a gradual release of energy, keeping blood sugar levels stable. Athletes engaged in endurance sports like cycling or running benefit from the sustainable energy quinoa provides.

BLUEBERRIES: Blueberries are rich in antioxidants, especially compounds called anthocyanins. These antioxidants help combat the damage from free radicals that can occur during intense and prolonged physical exercise. Blueberries are ideal for endurance athletes, such as triathletes, as they can reduce the risk of muscle fatigue and promote better recovery.

MACA: Maca is known for its adaptogenic properties, which can help the body adapt to stress, including physical stress related to training. This superfood is particularly useful for athletes experiencing intense training periods or participating in endurance competitions. Maca can contribute to improved endurance and overall energy.

CHIA SEEDS: Chia seeds are loaded with fiber, protein, and omega-3 fatty acids. These small seeds can absorb a considerable amount of liquid, becoming gel-like, making them an ideal option for maintaining hydration during physical activity. Athletes training in hot or humid environments can benefit from including chia seeds in their diet.

Other valuable allies:

BANANAS: Bananas are a natural source of carbohydrates, potassium, and vitamins, especially vitamin B6. These nutrients are important for maintaining electrolyte balance and preventing muscle cramps during physical activity. Bananas are a convenient snack for athletes and can be consumed before or during training to support energy and endurance.

OATS: Oats are another food rich in complex carbohydrates, fiber, and protein. They provide a sustainable source of energy, helping to keep blood sugar levels stable. Endurance athletes, such as trail runners or long-distance swimmers, can benefit from including oats in their diet.

WALNUTS: Walnuts, hazelnuts, almonds, and other types of walnuts are rich in healthy fats, protein, and fiber. These portable snacks are perfect for athletes on the go. The fats in walnuts provide slow-release energy, which can be valuable for endurance activities like hiking.

HONEY: Honey is a natural source of simple sugars like glucose and fructose, which can be rapidly used as fuel during intense physical activity. It is a good option for athletes who need a quick energy boost, such as during a cycling race or marathon.

SUPERFOODS FOR MUSCLE REPAIR AND GROWTH

Muscle repair is a fundamental process for athletes seeking to improve their strength and performance. Do you engage in weightlifting or are you in a mass-building phase? Here are some superfoods that promote muscle repair and growth:

WILD SALMON: This fish is an excellent source of high-quality proteins and omega-3 fatty acids. Proteins provide the amino acids needed for muscle protein synthesis, while omega-3s can reduce post-workout muscle inflammation.

SACHA INCHI: Known as the "Inca peanut," this small nut is rich in omega-3 fatty acids, protein, and vitamin E. It is an excellent choice for athletes looking to support muscle growth and tissue repair.

SPINACH: Spinach is rich in iron, calcium, and vitamin K, essential nutrients for muscle and bone health.

Additionally, it contains nitrates that can improve oxygen utilization efficiency during physical activity.

WALNUTS: Nuts are a good source of protein, vitamin E, and antioxidants. They are an ideal snack for athletes looking to maintain their protein intake during training.

SPIRULINA: Spirulina is primarily composed of high-quality proteins, with a concentration ranging from 50% to 70% of its dry weight. These proteins contain all the essential amino acids needed for muscle protein synthesis. It is particularly useful as a protein supplement for vegetarians and vegans. Furthermore, the essential fatty acids found in spirulina, such as gamma-linolenic acid (GLA), can help reduce muscle inflammation after exercise, accelerating the recovery process and allowing for more frequent and intense training.

Other valuable allies:

EGGS: Eggs are one of the best sources of complete proteins, as they contain all essential amino acids required for muscle protein synthesis. They are also rich in B-group vitamins, such as B12, which is important for muscle cell formation.

WHITE MEATS: White meats contain all essential amino acids that the body cannot produce on its own and must obtain from the diet. These amino acids are particularly important for promoting muscle protein synthesis and optimal recovery after training. White meats tend to have significantly lower saturated fat content compared to red meats. Finally, the selenium they contain plays an important role as an antioxidant in the body, helping protect cells from free radical damage. During intensive training, the body can produce free radicals that contribute to muscle inflammation and oxidative damage.

TOFU: Tofu is rich in plant-based proteins and contains all essential amino acids. It is a popular choice for vegetarian and vegan athletes to support muscle growth.

Please note that a balanced diet that includes a variety of foods from different categories can provide a comprehensive range of nutrients essential for overall health and sports performance. Additionally, individual nutritional needs may vary, so it's advisable to consult with a sports nutritionist or dietitian to create a personalized nutrition plan based on your specific goals and requirements.

SUPERFOODS FOR WEIGHT MANAGEMENT

For athletes, maintaining the right body weight is crucial to optimize performance, not to mention that during certain phases of preparation, weight needs to be managed. Here are the superfoods that can play a key role in weight management, primarily due to their ability to provide a sense of satiety:

BLACK CABBAGE (KALE): This leafy green vegetable is rich in fiber and nutrients but relatively low in calories. Fiber contributes to a feeling of fullness, making it ideal for athletes looking to maintain a healthy body weight.

QUINOA: This whole grain is rich in protein and fiber. Proteins, like fiber, help maintain satiety. Additionally, quinoa has a low glycemic index, which means it doesn't cause spikes in blood sugar, aiding appetite control.

AVOCADO: Avocados are a source of healthy monounsaturated fats. These fats, along with fiber and protein, can help reduce hunger and improve the feeling of fullness. Always pay attention to portion sizes as avocados are calorie-dense.

CHIA SEEDS: In addition to maintaining stable energy levels, as mentioned, these small seeds are rich in fiber and can absorb a significant amount of liquid, forming a gel in the stomach that increases satiety.

GREEN TEA: Green tea is known for its thermogenic properties, which can help burn calories more efficiently. It is also rich in antioxidants and can support metabolism.

Other valuable allies:

LEAFY GREEN VEGETABLES: Vegetables like spinach, kale, and lettuce are rich in fiber and water, making them very filling. They have a low-calorie content, meaning you can consume large quantities without introducing many calories. You can use them as a base for salads, add them to soups, or blend them into smoothies.

PUMPKINS & ZUCCHINIS: These vegetables are low in calories but packed with fiber and water. They can be used in many recipes to reduce the overall calorie intake of the meal.

BERRIES: Strawberries, blueberries, raspberries, and other berries are rich in fiber and antioxidants. They are sweet and satisfying but have fewer calories compared to many other fruits.

SUPERFOODS FOR RECOVERY AND REDUCING INFLAMMATION

After intense training, the body needs to recover and combat inflammation. Providing the right nutrients at this stage is particularly helpful in shortening recovery times. Some superfoods that can aid in this process include:

TURMERIC: This spice contains curcumin, known for its anti-inflammatory properties. It can be consumed as a supplement or added to various preparations (both dishes and smoothies) to help reduce post-workout inflammation.

WILD SALMON: In addition to being a good source of protein, wild salmon contains omega-3 fatty acids that have anti-inflammatory properties. It is an excellent food to include in your post-workout diet.

NATTO: This fermented soy-based product is rich in vitamin K2 and probiotics, which assist in managing intestinal inflammation, which can affect recovery and overall well-being.

Other valuable allies:

GINGER: The gingerol in ginger is known for its anti-inflammatory properties. You can add freshly grated ginger to tea or smoothies, or use it to flavor your dishes.

CHILI PEPPERS: The capsaicin in spicy peppers has been shown to have anti-inflammatory effects. If you can tolerate spicy food, you can add chili peppers to your meals for a burst of flavor and health benefits.

OATS: Oats are a source of soluble fiber called beta-glucans, which can help reduce inflammation. They are a healthy option for a post-workout snack.

SUPERFOODS FOR MENTAL WELLNESS AND EMOTIONAL BALANCE

Mental health and concentration are crucial for sports performance and overall well-being. Some superfoods that promote emotional well-being include:

GREEN TEA: Green tea contains catechins, known antioxidants, which can have positive effects on mental health. They can contribute to improving mood and concentration.

DARK CHOCOLATE: In moderate amounts, dark chocolate contains antioxidants and can have heart and mood-related benefits. Cocoa is known to stimulate the production of endorphins, the "feel-good" neurotransmitters.

GOJI BERRIES: These berries are rich in antioxidants and vitamin C, which can support brain health and the immune system. They are often consumed dried as snacks or added to smoothies and yogurt.

YACON: Yacon is rich in inulin, a prebiotic that can support gut health. A healthy gut is often associated with better emotional balance.

SPINACH: Spinach is rich in folates, which can support brain function and have a positive impact on mood.

Other valuable allies:

BRAZIL NUTS: These nuts are one of the best dietary sources of selenium, a mineral that can play a role in mood regulation.

PUMPKIN SEEDS: Pumpkin seeds are rich in magnesium, which is associated with improved mood and stress management.

CHICKPEAS: Chickpeas are a good source of tryptophan, an amino acid precursor to serotonin. These legumes can contribute to mood improvement.

SUPERFOODS FOR CARDIOVASCULAR HEALTH

Athletes must pay attention to cardiovascular health to ensure that the heart and circulatory system are in excellent condition. Some superfoods that promote cardiovascular health include:

ACAI: Its richness in antioxidants, especially anthocyanins, and omega-3 fatty acids can help reduce the risk of heart disease.

SPIRULINA: Studies have suggested that spirulina can help lower LDL cholesterol ("bad cholesterol") and improve artery health.

GREEK YOGURT: Calcium, found in good amounts in Greek yogurt, plays an important role in muscle contraction, including the heart's. Maintaining adequate levels of calcium in the body is important for cardiovascular well-being. Additionally, compared to many dairy products, Greek yogurt tends to be lower in saturated fats, which are associated with an increased risk of heart disease. Finally, the antioxidants and vitamins, such as vitamin B12, found in Greek yogurt are important for cardiovascular and overall health.

Other valuable allies:

APPLES: Apples are rich in fiber and antioxidants, which can help reduce the risk of heart disease. The classic "an apple a day keeps the doctor away" saying holds true!

GARLIC: Garlic is known for its heart-healthy properties, including its ability to lower blood pressure and reduce cholesterol.

BARLEY: Barley is a source of beta-glucans, similar to those in oats, which can help lower cholesterol and improve artery health.

SUPERFOODS FOR JOINT AND BONE HEALTH

Joint and bone health is crucial for all athletes who often put stress on their joints. Some superfoods that support joint and bone health include:

TURMERIC: Curcumin, the active compound in turmeric, is a potent natural anti-inflammatory. It can help reduce joint inflammation and has been studied for its potential in arthritis treatment.

WILD SALMON: In addition to supporting muscle repair with omega-3s, wild salmon can reduce joint inflammation and support bone health.

BLACK CABBAGE (KALE): Black cabbage provides a double benefit for bone health: calcium for structure (calcium is a major component of bones) and vitamin K for metabolism. Vitamin K plays a critical role in bone health. Specifically, vitamin K2 is involved in regulating bone metabolism: it helps direct calcium into bones, preventing it from accumulating in arteries or other unwanted areas of the body. This can help reduce the risk of calcifications and promote cardiovascular health.

Other valuable allies:

GINGER: Gingerol, the active compound in ginger, can help reduce joint inflammation and may be useful for people with arthritis.

WALNUTS: Walnuts contain omega-3 fatty acids, manganese, and copper, all nutrients that can support joint and bone health.

SESAME: Sesame is rich in calcium, magnesium, copper, and zinc. These minerals are important for bone mineralization and joint health.

Well, that was a chapter with a lot of information. You must have noticed that some superfoods fulfill multiple functions - that's why they're super.

I hope these broad categories have helped you focus on your main needs: learning to create a targeted dietary strategy for one or more specific requirements.

Now, what's missing is something fundamental - how to incorporate these superfoods into your daily routine. Let's see how.

7.

DIETARY NEEDS THROUGHOUT VARIOUS TRAINING PHASES

Choosing superfoods and the right foods based on your specific sports needs is the most complex aspect because requirements change, and so should your diet. I might sound repetitive, but I must emphasize this essential concept: when it comes to incorporating superfoods into your diet, there's no one-size-fits-all solution that remains unchanged over time. Your needs are ever-evolving and differ from those of another athlete, influencing the selection of foods to include in your daily diet. The "challenge" lies in planning your diet to align with your current needs.

Do you know you have an important competition in a month? Well, the grocery list for the first week will be different from the next three weeks because as you approach the competition, your dietary requirements will change.

The key to effective use of superfoods in sports is adaptability. Just as you vary your workouts, you should also vary and adapt your diet.

Understanding what your body requires during different training phases allows you to plan which nutrients to prioritize. Let's simplify by discussing the phases typically encountered in sports preparation.

MUSCLE MASS GAIN PHASE

During the period when your goal is to gain muscle mass, your nutritional strategy should include high-protein foods rich in amino acids, the essential nutrients your muscles need to grow and repair. Let's delve into the requirements of this phase.

High-Quality Proteins: Proteins are the fundamental building blocks for muscle construction. Superfoods rich in proteins are the starting point for those aiming to increase muscle mass. Among these, wild salmon stands out for its excellence. This fish provides high-quality proteins essential for muscle protein synthesis. Furthermore, salmon is rich in amino acids, including leucine, which plays a crucial role in stimulating muscle growth.

Omega-3 Fatty Acids: In addition to proteins, wild salmon is also an extraordinary source of omega-3 fatty acids, known for their numerous health benefits. Omega-3s can play a key role in muscle growth in various ways:

- **Reducing Inflammation**: Omega-3 fatty acids have anti-inflammatory properties that can contribute to reducing chronic inflammation, creating a favorable environment for muscle growth.

- **Improving Insulin Sensitivity**: Omega-3s can improve insulin sensitivity, allowing better nutrient uptake by muscle cells. This can promote the transport of amino acids needed for muscle protein synthesis.

- **Promoting Anabolism**: Omega-3s can positively influence muscle anabolism, stimulating muscle protein synthesis and reducing muscle breakdown.

Leucine: Leucine, a branched-chain amino acid (BCAA), deserves special mention when it comes to muscle mass gain. This amino acid has been shown to play a key role in stimulating muscle protein synthesis. Wild salmon is a source of leucine, but you can also find it in eggs, chicken, and tofu. All these foods play a crucial role in muscle anabolism.

Examples of Superfoods and Preferred Foods in this Phase: wild salmon, quinoa, spinach, walnuts and almonds, tofu, Greek yogurt, lean meats, eggs.

STRENGTH OR ENDURANCE ENHANCEMENT PHASE

Improving strength and endurance is a key goal for many athletes. A proper energy reserve allows you to endure intense and prolonged workouts.

Complex Carbohydrates: Superfoods like quinoa are known for being rich in complex carbohydrates, providing a slow-release energy source. This means they offer a constant and sustained source of fuel for your body during extended workouts. Here's how complex carbohydrates can help improve your strength and endurance:

- **Consistent Energy Supply**: During endurance workouts or prolonged weightlifting sessions, your body requires a constant supply of energy. Complex carbohydrates are gradually broken down, providing a steady release of glucose to the muscles, allowing you to sustain effort for a longer period.

- **Glycogen Reserve Preservation**: Complex carbohydrates help preserve your muscle and liver glycogen reserves. This is essential for extending your endurance during a workout, as glycogen reserves are a key source of energy.

- **Performance Enhancement**: Adequate intake of complex carbohydrates can enhance your sports performance, allowing you to tackle more intense workouts and maintain strength and endurance over a longer duration.

Examples of Superfoods and Preferred Foods in this Phase: In addition to quinoa, you can support your strength and endurance during training by including bananas, walnuts and seeds, sweet potatoes, spinach, in your diet.

PRE-COMPETITION PREPARATION PHASE

The pre-competition phase is a critical time for both professionals and amateurs. In the days, weeks, or even months leading up to a specific competition, you build the outcome of your performance, at least the expected one. It's the period in which you can maximize your energy and endurance levels, ensuring that your body is ready to compete at its best.

Complex Carbohydrates: When preparing for a competition, one of your main goals is to ensure a constant supply of energy. As in the strength and endurance enhancement phase, superfoods rich in complex carbohydrates play a crucial role in providing a continuous release of energy:

- **Gradual Glucose Release**: Complex carbohydrates found in quinoa are slowly broken down in your digestive system, providing a constant release of glucose into your bloodstream. This means your body has access to a stable source of energy throughout your entire workout.

- **Sustaining Physical Activity**: Cereals like quinoa or oats are an ideal choice for athletes because they offer the energy needed to maintain high performance during intense physical activity.

Examples of Superfoods and Preferred Foods in this Phase: To be prepared for various scenarios, the approach to a competition involves a variety of workouts and dietary diversity. While quinoa is an exceptional superfood for energy, it's also essential to consider fresh fruits (e.g., grapes, rich in sugars, especially glucose, easily converted into energy; oranges, a source of carbohydrates and vitamin C), as well as leafy greens (spinach and Swiss chard, for instance, are packed with iron and other essential vitamins for muscle health) and proteins (as we know, salmon, chicken, turkey, and tofu).

COMPETITION PHASE

The competition day is the culmination of weeks or even months of training and preparation, and having a well-defined nutritional plan is crucial to ensure optimal performance. Nutritional requirements will vary greatly depending on the sport you practice, so it's essential to tailor your daily diet to the specific demands of your sport. To do this effectively, you need to:

Understand the Requirements of Your Sport Discipline. Here are some examples:

- Marathon or Long-Distance Running: In these disciplines, energy is crucial, and complex carbohydrates like whole grain pasta, rice, and sweet potatoes can provide a long-lasting energy source. The goal is to maintain a constant blood glucose level to avoid fatigue.

- Weightlifting or Strength Sports: Athletes practicing strength sports like weightlifting require an adequate amount of protein for explosive strength and muscle recovery. Lean protein sources like chicken, fish, and eggs may be prioritized.

- Team Sports: In sports like soccer or basketball, energy is important, but it's also crucial to maintain endurance and focus. A combination of carbohydrates, proteins, and healthy fats is often recommended.
- Water Sports: Athletes engaged in water sports, such as swimming, may have particularly high hydration needs. Adequate hydration and electrolyte supplementation, when necessary, are essential.

Plan the Right Timing for Meals and Snacks: Once you understand the requirements of your sport discipline, you can plan meals based on the competition time. It's crucial not to arrive too depleted or, conversely, with ongoing digestion. For example:

- Breakfast: You might opt for a breakfast rich in complex carbohydrates if you practice a high-endurance discipline. Oatmeal with fruit and walnuts can be an excellent choice.
- Lunch: If you have an afternoon competition, lunch should be light but nourishing. A serving of grilled chicken with vegetables and brown rice could be a balanced choice.

- Snacks: Snacks like walnuts, Greek yogurt with fruit, or a protein bar can be useful between meals (or as a substitute for lunch if the competition is in the late morning) to maintain the right energy levels.

- Post-Competition: After the competition, it's important to replenish energy reserves and promote muscle recovery. Water, electrolytes, and a snack combining carbohydrates and proteins can be an appropriate choice.

As you can see, each phase of your preparation requires the support of dedicated foods. Superfoods often come to the aid of one or more phases: what you need to do now is finally plan a series of meals that introduce these allies based on the training period you are in.

Now that you have this information, let's go ahead and prepare the shopping list.

8.

EFFECTIVE SHOPPING LISTS FOR YOUR NEEDS

Now that you have a strategy in mind and know your functional foods, it's time to put a dietary training plan into action.

It all starts with a well-crafted shopping list. Once you've created a scheme, a strategy, you can focus on your days without worrying about food.

Firstly, let's look at the characteristics a good shopping list should have:

- **Regular:** Planning your weekly shopping list is the first step towards controlling your diet. The weekly list ensures you always have fresh foods available and allows you to plan meals for the entire week, considering the training and recovery needs of that time. For instance, if you expect an intense week of training, you can include suitable superfoods to maintain high energy levels. In addition to the weekly list, you will have a monthly (or even quarterly) shopping list for foods you consume less frequently or that have a longer shelf life, ensuring you always have them on hand to mix and match with fresh ones.

- **Varied:** Variety is key to receiving a complete range of essential nutrients. By including a wide variety of superfoods in your shopping list, you can cover a broad spectrum of nutrients such as proteins, carbohydrates, healthy fats, vitamins, and minerals. For example, you can alternate between different protein sources like lean meat, fish, legumes, and tofu to ensure you get all the essential amino acids.

- **Seasonal:** In addition to the positive impact on the environment and your wallet, seasonal superfoods and foods are a wise choice in terms of taste and nutrition. When you purchase seasonal products, you are guaranteed to get fresh foods at their peak nutritional quality. An example is ripe tomatoes in the summer, which are not only delicious but also offer optimal levels of vitamin C and lycopene.

- **In Line with Your Training Phase:** To make your shopping list consistent, you need to plan it in advance and align it with the training phase you are currently in. Are you in a bulking phase? Prioritize certain superfoods. Need to recover after a race? Focus on recovery-supporting superfoods.

Now, let's get into the lists. The first piece of advice you can implement to have a perfect list is to create more than one. Start by categorizing superfoods and other foods based on their type, estimating average consumption, and indicating where you can easily purchase them. This way, you'll have everything under control: you'll know where and when to buy the foods you need.

We've already done some of the work for you! Below, you'll find foods categorized by type/frequency of purchase so you can place them on your weekly, monthly, or quarterly list. Keep in mind that quantities are influenced by various factors such as age, sex, weight, and training loads. We can't provide exact amounts, so here are indicative quantities that can serve as a guide:

Make sure to customize these quantities based on your individual needs and dietary preferences.

WEEKLY SHOPPING LIST

(Tear or take a photo!)

- Blueberries
- Black Cabbage
- Avocado
- Wild Salmon
- Eggs
- Spinach
- Apples
- Bananas
- Sweet Potatoes
- Zucchini
- Greek Yogurt
- Protein Curds
- Fresh Ginger
- Chicken or Turkey
- Fatty Fish (e.g., mackerel)
- Tofu
- Seasonal Fruits
- Seasonal Vegetables
- Sorrel (when available)
- Natto (when available)

MONTHLY SHOPPING LIST

(Tear or take a photo!)

- Brown Rice
- Quinoa
- Whole Wheat Pasta
- Barley
- Whole Wheat Crackers or Biscuits
- Flax Seeds
- Dark Chocolate
- Walnuts
- Peanuts
- Almonds
- Oat Flakes
- Sesame Seeds
- Canned Chickpeas
- Canned Legumes (e.g., lentils, beans)
- Extra Virgin Olive Oil
- Honey
- Green Tea
- Pumpkin Seeds
- Camelina Oil

QUARTERLY SHOPPING LIST

(Tear or take a photo!)

- Chia Seeds
- Acai Powder
- Spirulina Powder
- Baobab Powder
- Maca Powder
- Kelp Powder
- Camu Camu Powder
- Lucuma Powder
- Dried Yacón
- Baobab Powder (again)
- Roasted Sacha Inchi
- Amaranth (seeds or flour)
- Fenugreek (seeds or powder)
- Turmeric
- Chili Powder
- Garlic Powder

9.

CREATE YOUR WEEKLY SUPERMENU

Alright, you've done your shopping, and the fridge is fully stocked. It's time to head to the kitchen.

In this chapter, we'll create an example of a weekly sports menu. I want to give you concrete ideas so you can customize the menu based on your tastes and training phases, varying foods and carbohydrate and protein percentages as you like.

Some rules can help you when building your personalized menu.

In the menu below, I've divided each day into 6 meals:
- Breakfast
- Mid-morning snack
- Lunch
- Afternoon snack
- Dinner
- Evening snack

Each day's menu provides approximately 3,000 kcal, distributed as follows:
- Carbohydrates: about 45% of total calories
- Proteins: about 35% of total calories
- Fats: about 20% of total calories

The menu includes both fresh foods and long-term storage foods. Less common superfoods can be added as needed.

[MONDAY]

Breakfast
- Oatmeal with blueberries and walnuts
- One banana
- Green tea

Mid-morning Snack
- Cottage cheese with chia seeds

Lunch
- Black cabbage, avocado, and wild salmon salad
- Quinoa as a side dish
- One apple

Afternoon Snack
- Wild salmon on whole grain crackers

Dinner
- Grilled chicken with baked sweet potatoes and grilled zucchini
- Sautéed spinach with fresh garlic
- Green tea

Evening Snack
- Greek yogurt with walnuts

[TUESDAY]

Breakfast

- Smoothie with banana, spinach, Greek yogurt, and chia seeds
- Slice of whole wheat bread with avocado

Mid-morning Snack

- Sliced apples with almond butter

Lunch

- Quinoa salad with walnuts, sorrel, and tofu
- Protein curds as dessert

Afternoon Snack

- Baby carrots with hummus

Dinner

- Baked wild salmon with lemon and ginger sauce
- Brown rice as a side dish
- Grilled seasonal vegetables

Evening Snack

- Banana sorbet: freeze slices of ripe banana and blend with Greek yogurt and a sprinkle of maca powder

[WEDNESDAY]

Breakfast
- Banana and oat pancakes with blueberries
- One orange
- Matcha smoothie

Mid-morning Snack
- Greek yogurt with acai powder and walnuts

Lunch
- Spinach salad with grilled chicken and avocado
- Quinoa as a side dish
- One seasonal fruit

Afternoon Snack
- Almonds and raisins

Dinner
- Grilled tofu with baked sweet potatoes and grilled zucchini
- Sautéed black cabbage with fresh garlic

Evening Snack
- Avocado mousse with Greek yogurt and cocoa powder

[THURSDAY]

Breakfast
- Smoothie with banana, spinach, Greek yogurt, and chia seeds
- Slice of whole wheat bread with avocado

Mid-morning Snack
- Pears with Greek yogurt and acai powder

Lunch
- Quinoa salad with walnuts, sorrel, and tofu
- Protein curds as dessert

Afternoon Snack
- Baby carrots with hummus

Dinner
- Scrambled eggs with spinach and flax seeds
- Brown rice as a side dish
- Fresh seasonal vegetables

Evening Snack
- Greek yogurt with oats, lucuma powder, and walnuts

[FRIDAY]

Breakfast

- Oat and coconut pancakes with almond cream
- One hard-boiled egg
- Green tea

Mid-morning Snack

- Greek yogurt with baobab powder

Lunch

- Black cabbage salad with grilled chicken
- Barley as a side dish
- One seasonal fruit

Afternoon Snack

- Protein curds on whole grain crackers

Dinner

- Grilled tofu with baked sweet potatoes
- Sautéed black cabbage with ginger
- Ginger and lemon infusion

Evening Snack

- One seasonal fruit

[SATURDAY]

Breakfast
- Oatmeal with blueberries and walnuts
- One seasonal fruit
- Turmeric tea

Mid-morning Snack
- Greek yogurt with blueberries and chia seeds

Lunch
- Grilled turkey with avocado
- Quinoa as a side dish
- Apple for dessert

Afternoon Snack
- A handful of almonds and an apple

Dinner
- Grilled mackerel with grilled zucchini
- Chickpea hummus

Evening Snack
- Greek yogurt with honey and walnuts

[SUNDAY]

Breakfast
- Spirulina smoothie
- Slice of whole wheat bread with avocado
- Nuts

Mid-morning Snack
- A handful of peanuts and an apple

Lunch
- Sorrel and scrambled eggs on quinoa
- Protein curds as dessert

Afternoon Snack
- Greek yogurt with blueberries

Dinner
- Whole wheat pasta with wild salmon
- Grilled seasonal vegetables

Evening Snack
- Spirulina yogurt with pumpkin seeds

Want a few more recipes? Read the next chapter!

10.

RECIPES FEATURING SUPERFOODS

To vary your preparations, you can try some of the combinations I suggest. Here are some ideas divided by their level of preparation difficulty.

[SUPER EASY IDEAS]

Blueberry Greek Yogurt

Preparation Time: 5 minutes

Ingredients:

- 150 g Greek yogurt
- 30 g fresh blueberries
- 1 teaspoon honey
- 1 teaspoon chopped hazelnuts

Preparation:

- Mix fresh blueberries with Greek yogurt.
- Top with a handful of chopped hazelnuts and a drizzle of honey.

Salmon Bowl

Preparation Time: 15 minutes

Ingredients:

- 150-200 g fresh wild salmon
- 90 g black rice
- 80 g fresh spinach
- 1 teaspoon flax seeds
- Pinch of salt
- 1 tablespoon extra virgin olive oil

Preparation:

* Bring a large pot of salted water to a boil, add a garlic clove, and cook the black rice; drain and toss with a drizzle of extra virgin olive oil.
* In a hot non-stick skillet, cook the wild salmon, without adding seasonings, for about 3 minutes per side to achieve a nice Maillard reaction.
* In a sufficiently large bowl, layer the rice, fresh spinach leaves, and then the salmon. Garnish with a sprinkle of crushed flax seeds.

Banana & Acai Smoothie

Preparation Time: 5 minutes
Ingredients:

* 1 ripe banana
* 1 teaspoon acai powder
* 1 cup (about 240 ml) almond milk

Preparation:

* Blend the banana with almond milk until smooth, then add the acai powder and mix briefly.
* For extra freshness, you can add a couple of ice cubes while blending.
* Optionally garnish with a vanilla or licorice stick.

Quinoa Salad

Preparation Time: 10 minutes

Ingredients:

- 90 g quinoa
- 40 g fresh kale
- 20 g fresh ginger
- 1 tablespoon extra virgin olive oil

Preparation:

- Cook the quinoa according to the package instructions, usually in boiling salted water for about ten minutes, then let it cool with a drizzle of olive oil to prevent sticking.
- Mix with chopped kale and freshly grated ginger.
- Season with extra virgin olive oil and adjust the salt.

Maca Energy Bites

Preparation Time: 10 minutes

Ingredients:

- 100 g oat flakes
- 3 teaspoons maca powder
- 30 g walnuts

* 30 g raisins
* 2 tablespoons honey

Preparation:

* Crumble the walnuts, then in a sufficiently large bowl, mix all the ingredients.
* Adjust honey to thicken as desired and shape into small balls or bars.
* Chill them in the fridge before serving.

Dark Chocolate & Avocado Mousse

Preparation Time: 10 minutes

Ingredients:

* 1 ripe avocado
* 20 g dark chocolate
* 1 tablespoon honey

Preparation:

* Blend ripe avocado with dark chocolate and honey. Chill before serving as dessert.

Green Smoothie

Preparation Time: 5 minutes

Ingredients:

- ❖ 30 g fresh spinach
- ❖ 1 ripe banana
- ❖ 60 g Greek yogurt
- ❖ 1 teaspoon spirulina powder

Preparation:

- ❖ Blend everything, optionally adding one or two ice cubes, and enjoy as an energy-boosting snack.

Tropical Fruit Smoothie with Camu Camu

Preparation Time: 5 minutes

Ingredients:

- ❖ 1/2 ripe banana
- ❖ 1/2 mango
- ❖ 50 g pineapple
- ❖ 1 teaspoon camu camu powder
- ❖ 50 ml coconut milk

Preparation:

- ❖ Blend everything, optionally adding one or two ice cubes, and savor this exotic smoothie.

[EASY IDEAS]

Sautéed Tofu with Sorrel

Preparation Time: 15 minutes

Ingredients:

- 150 g tofu
- 30 g fresh sorrel
- 20 g fresh ginger
- 90 g quinoa
- 2 tablespoons extra virgin olive oil

Preparation:

- Cook quinoa according to package instructions, then drain and add a drizzle of extra virgin olive oil.
- In a skillet, sauté tofu with chopped sorrel.
- Plate it with quinoa at the base, then tofu, and garnish with freshly grated ginger.

Acai Bowl with Fresh Fruit

Preparation Time: 10 minutes

Ingredients:

- 1 banana
- 1 apple
- 30 g blueberries
- 50 ml almond milk
- 20 g baobab powder
- 10 g chia seeds

Preparation:

* Cut the banana and apple into small pieces.
* In a large bowl, add acai powder and almond milk and mix.
* Garnish with blueberries and chia seeds.

Wild Salmon in Curry

Preparation Time: 25 minutes

Ingredients:

* 150-200 g fresh wild salmon
* 15 g curry
* 90 g whole grain rice
* 30 g kale
* 10 g sesame seeds

Preparation:

* Sprinkle curry powder over the salmon on all sides, then bake in a preheated static oven at 180°C for about 20 minutes. Then switch on the grill at 240°C and finish cooking for another 3-4 minutes to create a crispy crust.
* Meanwhile, cook the rice in plenty of salted water with previously chopped kale.
* Plate it and sprinkle the rice with a handful of sesame seeds.

Tofu Scramble with Spinach

Preparation Time: 10 minutes
Ingredients:

- ❖ 150 g tofu
- ❖ 30 g spinach
- ❖ 1/4 teaspoon chili powder
- ❖ 1 tablespoon extra virgin olive oil

Preparation:

- ❖ Sauté diced tofu with spinach and chili powder.

[EXPERIMENTAL IDEAS]

Salmon Sashimi with Camu Camu Sauce

Preparation Time: 15 minutes
Ingredients:

- ❖ 100 g raw wild salmon fillet
- ❖ 15 g camu camu powder
- ❖ 20 ml low-sodium soy sauce
- ❖ 20 g fresh ginger

Preparation:

- ❖ Slice the wild salmon fillet into thin slices and place it on a cold plate.

❖ Prepare a sauce by mixing camu camu powder, soy sauce, and freshly grated ginger.

Amaranth Risotto with Spinach and Walnuts

Preparation Time: 45 minutes

Ingredients:

❖ 90 g amaranth
❖ 1 shallot
❖ 25 g butter or 30 ml extra virgin olive oil
❖ 150 g fresh spinach
❖ 30 g walnuts
❖ Vegetables for vegetable broth (1 potato, 1 carrot, 1 onion, celery, bay leaf)

Preparation:

❖ First, prepare the vegetable broth in a large pot: fill it with about 1 liter of water, then add the potato, carrot, onion, some celery ribs, and a bay leaf. Bring it all to a boil and let it cook over medium-low heat for about 20 minutes. Strain the broth to separate the vegetables from the other ingredients. Keep the broth warm.
❖ In a non-stick skillet, melt the butter (or heat the extra virgin olive oil for a lighter version) over medium heat. Add finely chopped shallot and

sauté until it becomes translucent, which should take about 2-3 minutes.

* Add the amaranth to the skillet and toast it for about 1-2 minutes, stirring constantly. This will help develop the flavor of the amaranth.

* Add warm vegetable broth, one ladle at a time, stirring constantly, and wait until the liquid is completely absorbed before adding the next ladle of broth. Continue this process until the amaranth is cooked, about 15-20 minutes (I suggest checking the time indicated on the package).

* Meanwhile, heat a separate skillet and toast the chopped walnuts until they become slightly golden and fragrant. Set them aside.

* When the amaranth is almost done, add roughly chopped fresh spinach and mix well until they shrink in volume, then remove the skillet from the heat and add the toasted walnuts.

* Serve the hot amaranth risotto, optionally garnishing it with some fresh spinach leaves or extra chopped walnuts if desired.

Natto and Curry Eggs

Preparation Time: 40 minutes

Ingredients:

* 50 g natto
* 2 eggs
* 1 teaspoon curry powder
* 90 g whole grain rice
* Salt and pepper to taste
* 15 ml soy sauce
* 15 ml extra virgin olive oil

Preparation:

* Start by cooking whole grain rice according to package instructions.
* Put the natto in a bowl, then add soy sauce (or the natto sauce included in the package), mix well until the natto becomes slightly sticky, and the sauce is well incorporated. Cover the bowl and set it aside.
* In another small bowl, mix curry powder with a little water to create a curry paste. Ensure you get a smooth, lump-free consistency.
* In a non-stick skillet, heat some extra virgin olive oil over medium heat. Add beaten eggs with a pinch of salt and pepper and slowly stir until they start to set but are still soft. At this point, add the curry paste you prepared earlier and mix well to distribute it evenly among the eggs. Continue

cooking for a couple of minutes until the eggs are cooked, and the curry sauce is fragrant.

* Using a cookie cutter, plate the whole grain rice, then lay the natto on top. Finally, place the curry eggs on top of the natto, garnishing with your choice of fresh herbs (e.g., cilantro or parsley) or finely chopped scallions if desired.

Lucuma Pastries

Preparation Time: 60 minutes
Ingredients:
* 6 whole grain cookies
* 1-2 tablespoons lucuma powder (depending on your taste)
* 55 g dark chocolate

Preparation:
* Start by preparing the base for the pastries. Finely chop the whole grain cookies until you get compact crumbs. You can do this by placing the cookies in a resealable plastic bag and crushing them with a rolling pin or using a food processor. Transfer the mixture to a bowl. Add lucuma powder and mix well until you have a uniform mixture.

* Now create the first layer. Prepare a square or rectangular mold, usually lined with parchment paper or lightly greased with a little oil. Evenly distribute half of the cookie and lucuma crumbs on the bottom of the mold. Use the back of a spoon or a glass to compact the mixture into an even layer. Set aside some of the mixture.

* Melt the dark chocolate in a double boiler or in the microwave, stirring occasionally until completely smooth, then pour the layer of melted chocolate over the first layer of cookie and lucuma. Ensure that the chocolate layer is even.

* Sprinkle the remaining cookie and lucuma crumbs over the top. Gently press with the back of a spoon to make the crumbs adhere.

* Let it cool in the refrigerator for at least 30 minutes or until the chocolate has solidified completely. Once cooled, you can remove the entire block from the edges of the mold and cut it into squares or rectangles, depending on your desired size.

I'm sure your experiments have brought you satisfaction; now you can share these superb dishes with your friends!

11.

CONCLUSIONS

Thank you for reading this far. We've come to the end of this short but intense journey through the fascinating world of superfoods.

In this little book, we've taken quite a ride: we've explored the fundamentals of superfoods, delved into the most famous ones, and unearthed the lesser-known ones. We've also talked about those that "didn't make it" but can still provide us with good satisfaction.

In these pages, you've seen how superfoods can contribute to improving your athletic performance, whether you're a dedicated marathon runner or an evening jog enthusiast.

In the chapters dedicated to shopping lists and weekly menus, I've tried to simplify your life because, yes, wandering around the supermarket without a clear plan can be stressful. Finally, the recipes: I hope you've already tried at least one of them.

In closing, I say to you: never stop raising the bar, informing yourself and exploring, discovering and experimenting, in both nutrition and sports. Every time you learn something new, you're simply better than before.

If you enjoyed this book or found it helpful, please consider leaving a review on Amazon. I would greatly appreciate it!

www.ingramcontent.com/pod-product-compliance
Lightning Source LLC
Chambersburg PA
CBHW050818260726
48660CB00004B/1503